DIABETES

DIABETES

The Biography

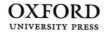

Robert Tattersall

OXFORD
UNIVERSITY PRESS

OXFORD
UNIVERSITY PRESS

Great Clarendon Street, Oxford OX2 6DP

Oxford University Press is a department of the University of Oxford.
It furthers the University's objective of excellence in research, scholarship,
and education by publishing worldwide in

Oxford New York

Auckland Cape Town Dar es Salaam Hong Kong Karachi
Kuala Lumpur Madrid Melbourne Mexico City Nairobi
New Delhi Shanghai Taipei Toronto

With offices in

Argentina Austria Brazil Chile Czech Republic France Greece
Guatemala Hungary Italy Japan Poland Portugal Singapore
South Korea Switzerland Thailand Turkey Ukraine Vietnam

Oxford is a registered trade mark of Oxford University Press
in the UK and in certain other countries

Published in the United States
by Oxford University Press Inc., New York

British Library Cataloguing in Publication Data
Data available

Library of Congress Cataloging-in-Publication Data
Tattersall, Robert, 1943–
Diabetes : the biography / Robert Tattersall.
p. ; cm.—(Biographies of disease)
Includes bibliographical references and index.
ISBN 978-0-19-954136-2 (hardback)
1. Diabetes—History. I. Title. II. Series: Biographies of disease (Oxford, England)
[DNLM: 1. Diabetes Mellitus—history. 2. History, Modern 1601-. WK
11.1 T221d 2009]
RC660.T38 2009
616.4'62—dc22 2009026413

Typeset by SPI Publisher Services, Pondicherry, India
Printed in Great Britain
on acid-free paper by
Clays Ltd, St Ives plc

ISBN 978-0-19-954136-2

PREFACE

I have long had an interest in medical history, and this increased when I spent three months at the Wellcome Institute for the History of Medicine in 1993. Its library (free to anyone) has been invaluable in my research, as have the porters at the Greenfield Library of Nottingham University Medical School, who have cheerfully descended into the bowels of the earth to retrieve dusty journals for me.

When I retired from clinical practice in 1998, my intention was (and still is) to write a definitive, exhaustively referenced, history of diabetes, which would be of interest primarily to doctors. However, I jumped at the suggestion of the editors of this series at Oxford University Press that I should write a biography of diabetes that would be about a tenth of the length of a full history with a minimum of references, for a wide general readership.

During the 1980s the British Diabetic Association (now Diabetes UK) decided to ban the use of diabetic as a noun. In this book I often talk about diabetics for two reasons: first, because it becomes tedious to keep reading about 'persons with diabetes' or 'diabetic people'. The other reason is that for most of the period I am writing about it was normal to use 'diabetic' as a noun.

Many of my friends in the world of diabetes have helped with my historical research, but I am particularly grateful to Edwin Gale, Harry Keen, Carl-Erik Mogensen, David McCulloch, and the late Michael Berger.

I also thank Bill and Helen Bynum, who have made many helpful suggestions and have constantly reminded me that I am not writing an article for the *Lancet*.

My wife, Bridget, has been a constant support and has made many valuable suggestions.

ROBERT TATTERSALL
Nottingham, 2009.

CONTENTS

LIST OF ILLUSTRATIONS

PROLOGUE

When people are asked to rank diseases in order of seriousness, diabetes is usually at the mild end of the spectrum. A journalist whose 16-year-old son had just been diagnosed wrote that he had always thought of it as 'something manageable and unprofound, a disease where not much happens'.[1] By contrast, a patient of mine who had had it for many years compared it to living with a tiger, since, as he said: 'If you look after it, and never turn your back on it, you can live with a tiger. If you neglect it, it will pounce on you and rip you to shreds.' The seriousness of the disease was officially recognized in 2006, when the General Assembly of the United Nations described diabetes as 'a chronic, debilitating and costly disease associated with severe complications, which poses severe risks for families, states and the entire world'.[2]

Diabetes, or, to give it its scientific name, *diabetes mellitus*, is a disease in which the defining abnormality is an excessively high level of glucose (often just called sugar) in the blood. The cardinal symptoms in the young are an increased volume of urine (polyuria), thirst (polydipsia), and weight loss. There may also be excessive appetite (polyphagia), so that American doctors talk about patients having 'the polys'—polydipsia, polyuria, and polyphagia. Those who develop diabetes in middle or old age have less dramatic or no symptoms and may be diagnosed on a routine blood or urine test.

The simplicity of the diagnostic tests conceals the fact that diabetes is a complicated biochemical disorder that affects the metabolism of all components of our diet. Meals are broken down in the intestine into their component parts of fats (lipids), proteins (amino acids), and carbohydrates (which include sugars such as glucose) by enzymes produced in the pancreas, which lies behind the stomach and is known to butchers as sweetbread. The pancreas is a double organ. The exocrine (externally secreting) part, which forms 99 per cent of its bulk, produces enzymes, which are discharged into the duodenum. The endocrine (internally secreting) part of the pancreas consists of clusters of cells (the islets of Langerhans), which are scattered throughout the organ like islands in a sea. What determines whether glucose is burned immediately or stored in the liver or muscles is the hormone insulin, which is produced in the islets of Langerhans. Absence of insulin or resistance to its action causes diabetes.

Diabetes is not a single disease but a syndrome with at least fifty possible causes. However, there are two main types. In one, most common in children and young people, the insulin-producing cells of the islets (beta cells) are destroyed by anti-bodies made in the body (autoimmunity), and this eventually results in a complete absence of insulin. This condition used to be called juvenile or insulin-dependent diabetes, but is now called type 1.

The other form mainly affects people over the age of 40 and used to be called adult-onset, maturity-onset, or non-insulin-dependent diabetes. It is now called type 2 and is by far the most common type. In type 2, the beta cells are intact and, at least in the first few years, produce more insulin than normal because the target tissues (liver and fat) are resistant to its action.

In the healthy body the normal level of glucose in the blood is tightly maintained between 3.5 and 8 mmol/l (63–144 mg/dl).[3] Exposure to persistently high levels of glucose for many years damages small blood vessels, causing the long-term diabetic complications affecting the eyes (retinopathy), nerves (neuropathy), and kidneys (nephropathy). It is important to realize that diabetes is not just a glucose disease. There are also abnormalities of fat metabolism, which contribute to hardening of large arteries (atherosclerosis), causing heart attacks, strokes, and gangrene of the feet.

I have spent most of my working life looking after patients with, and researching, diabetes. It has been an absorbing journey. As the Birmingham physician John Malins wrote in his 1968 textbook:

> The more diabetic patients one sees the more difficult it becomes to present the simple picture that so many readers like. Diabetes is a disorder of such infinite variety that it becomes impossible to say that this always occurs or that never happens...today a diabetic clinic provides the widest clinical range of any speciality in medicine with metabolic, vascular, neurological and psychiatric problems outstanding. In addition there is a chance to enjoy some of the pleasures of general practice which arise from long acquaintance with many of the patients. The chance, all too frequent, to ease the last years of those whose health is slowly failing calls for all the resources of the general physician.[4]

The effects of diabetes are indeed highly variable, as the following examples show.

3

Identical twins with type 1 diabetes

In 1971, while doing research on diabetes in identical twins, I met Jane and Sandra, who were born in 1938. At age 5, when Jane developed diabetes, they were as alike as 'two peas in a pod'. Sandra has remained unaffected, a not uncommon situation for type 1 diabetes in identical twins, indicating that it is not purely a genetic disease. Being a child with diabetes is often lonely and stigmatizing (Fig. 1). Jane's glucose control was always poor and she had frequent hospital admissions as a teenager. This chronic ill health affected her development, so that her adult height was 2½ inches shorter than Sandra's and she started her periods four years later—healthy identical twins are the same height and start their periods in the same week or month. In her late teens Jane had anorexia nervosa and told me that she

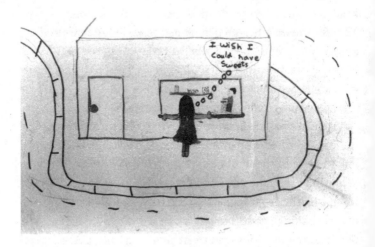

1. A child's drawing showing the loneliness of having diabetes.

deliberately underdosed herself with insulin to lose weight. She married in her 20s and, after three miscarriages, she had a still-born child. The first signs of diabetic eye damage were noted when she was 26, and by the age of 35 she was blind. Protein in her urine, the earliest sign of kidney damage, appeared when she was 24, and she was about to start dialysis when she died of a heart attack aged 37.

Before the first clinical use of insulin in 1922–3 Jane would have died within six months of diagnosis. What insulin did was to transform her illness from an acute rapidly fatal condition into a chronic one with what were eventually fatal complications. They are by no means inevitable, as shown by the next case.

Uncomplicated type 1 diabetes

In January 1931, Herbert, the 12-year-old son of a butcher in a small town near Nottingham, began to be increasingly thirsty. Things came to a head when he had to leave his confirmation service abruptly to 'have a wee'. After diabetes was diagnosed by his general practitioner (GP), he was admitted to hospital and discharged two weeks later on 5 units of insulin twice daily and a diet of only 35 grams of carbohydrate per day (equivalent to a small slice of bread). So little aftercare was provided that when the insulin he had been given was running low, his elder brother had to write to the local newspaper to ask where to get more. While in hospital he had to buy a syringe and urine testing kit. Later, when he broke his syringe (a regular occurrence as a result of daily boiling), he had to buy a new one for 5 shillings, 'a hell of a lot of money for me in those days' (£11 today). As a grow-ing boy he could not manage on so little carbohydrate and, in his late teens, broke the diet regularly and ate sweets. He had not been told that he could increase the dose of insulin and in 1939, after developing blurred vision, he went to the Eye Hospital, where he was told 'your eyes will never get better unless you take more care of your diabetes'. He was referred to a physician, who admitted him to hospital for seven weeks, after which he was discharged on a diet of 280 grams of carbohydrate and three doses of insulin a day. Surprisingly, after his next appointment in 1939, he was told not to come again, because 'you know how to take care of yourself.' He didn't really, but in 1941 he got married, and his wife Elsie bought a patient handbook, *The Diabetic ABC* by Dr R. D. Lawrence, which they used in lieu of a doctor for the next forty years. Herbert and Elsie lived above the butcher's shop, which Herbert took over from his father. Meals were always rigidly on time and Elsie tested his urine before every meal and weighed his food. The only alarms were that once or twice a year Herbert would become unconscious from low blood sugar during the night and Elsie would have to revive him. In 1981 the couple were surprised to be told by their GP, whom they had hardly ever seen, except for the childhood ailments of their children, that Herbert had to attend the hospital to be changed to a new strength of insulin. It was then that I met Herbert and was delighted to discover that, after fifty years, he had no diabetic complications. When I congratulated him, he said, 'That's the wife's doing. I wouldn't have managed without her.'

Type 2 or 'mild' diabetes

I took over the diabetic clinic in Nottingham in 1975 and three years later met Lilian, an overweight 60-year-old woman who was on tablets for diabetes. She had had sugar in her urine during her last pregnancy in 1957 but was well until 1963, when genital itching (*pruritus vulvae*) led to a diagnosis of diabetes. She attended the clinic for two years but was then sent back to her GP with a letter that read: 'I am discharging this lady with mild maturity onset diabetes back to your care.' She continued to collect her tablets but had no other supervision. When I met her after she had had diabetes for eighteen years she was blind, had had a heart attack, and had had one leg amputated below the knee. The reason for the referral to me was an ulcer on her remaining foot, which would not heal. Although complications in type 2 diabetes can be as serious or even worse than in type 1, it was often referred to as mild diabetes, probably the only example of a disease where the seriousness is determined by the perceived unpleasantness of the treatment—injections versus tablets.

Someone whose course is not dissimilar to that of Lilian is Sue Townsend (b. 1946), author of the Adrian Mole books. She developed diabetes at the age of 38 and after only fifteen years was blind from retinopathy and wheelchair bound because of a Charcot foot, a condition in which the ankle disintegrates as a result of nerve damage. Neuropathy has also destroyed the nerve endings in her fingers, so that, like most other blind diabetics, she cannot read Braille. She blames her complications on the fact that she cavalierly disregarded the disease and kept her blood sugars high to avoid the inconvenience of hypoglycaemic (low-blood-sugar) attacks.

A new kind of diabetes: MODY

As John Malins pointed out, diabetes is so variable that one can never say that 'this always occurs or that never happens'. When I was a medical student, it was axiomatic that normal-weight young people with diabetes needed insulin. Jennifer, whom I met in 1971, disproved that. She developed diabetes in 1943 at the age of 12, presenting with thirst and increased urination. She was put on insulin, but discontinued it on her own initiative between 1948 and 1951. When she returned to the clinic in 1951, she was relatively well but had a high blood sugar. She was given a stern telling-off and restarted on injections. In 1970 she insisted on being tried on anti-diabetic tablets, and, to the surprise of the doctors, they worked. I asked why she had been so certain she could manage without insulin; her answer was that her aunt and cousin had both developed diabetes in their teens and been put on insulin, but had been able to stop it after thirty years. I found two other patients in the clinic at King's College Hospital with very similar histories. They also had family members with the same unusual form of diabetes. I described them in a paper entitled 'Mild familial diabetes with dominant inheritance' and in 1975, while working with Professor Fajans in Ann Arbor, Michigan, changed this to Maturity Onset Type Diabetes or MODY, a name that has stuck.[5] In the 1990s it was found that diabetes in these families was caused by single gene mutations, and it is now clear that MODY (of which there are five separate types) accounts for 1–2 per cent of all diabetes.

A plague of diabetes

In the first two decades of the twentieth century what we now call type 1 diabetes was a tragic but rare condition. It remained uncommon until the second half of the century, when in several Western countries the number of new cases per year doubled or trebled over a twenty-year period before apparently reaching a plateau. This sort of change suggests an environmental factor, although exactly what this factor might be has remained elusive.

Type 2 diabetes is predominantly a disease of older and fatter people and has become increasingly common as a result of increased life expectancy, urbanization, lifestyle changes, and population growth. In the year 2000 it was estimated that approximately 171 million people worldwide, or about 4.6 per cent of people in the age range 20–79, were affected. This figure conceals tremendous variations between countries and within the same ethnic group. For example, in the 1990s about 3 per cent of rural Chinese in mainland China had diabetes compared to 13 per cent of Chinese in Mauritius, where living standards were much higher. At the same time, a similar picture was seen among Asian Indians, where about 4 per cent of those in rural India were diabetic compared to 23 per cent of Indians living in Fiji or Leicester, England. An observer in 1900 would have been amazed by the magnitude of these figures but not by the concept that diabetes was a product of wealth, dietary change, and urbanization. A Victorian physician had even described diabetes as 'one of the penalties of advanced civilization'.[6]

I

THE PISSING EVIL
Defining the disease

The earliest description of what might be diabetes is in an Egyptian papyrus of 1500 BC. The entry consists of the single phrase 'a medicine to drive away the passing of too much urine'.[1] Frequency and retention with overflow are also mentioned, making it uncertain whether what is being described is an excessive volume of urine (polyuria) or excessively frequent urination (frequency) as from infection or a bladder stone.

The Hindu physician Sushruta, who is thought to have written in the sixth century BC, described a disease of honey urine. The diagnosis was made by tasting the urine or noting that ants congregated round it—the latter is still one of the commonest ways of diagnosing diabetes in Africa today. The disease was perceived by Sushruta to be most common in indolent, overweight, and gluttonous people and ran in families. Physical exercise and vegetables were the mainstays of treatment in the obese, while the lean, in whom the disease was regarded as more serious, were prescribed a nourishing diet.

It is said that the father of medicine, Hippocrates of Cos (460–370 BC), did not recognize diabetes. However, there are indirect references in the Hippocratic Corpus that may be allusions to it. In *The Epidemics* patients are described in whom the volume of urine is greatly in excess of the amount of fluid drunk, which in a hot climate is significant and cannot be explained by a urinary infection. There are also several references to 'watery urine', which is what the dilute urine in untreated diabetes looks like.[2]

The first description of the symptoms of diabetes was by Aretaeus, who lived during the second century AD in Cappadocia. He thought the word *diabetes*, apparently already in common use, came from the Greek word for a siphon. His clinical description is marvellously vivid:

> Diabetes is a wonderful affection, not very frequent among men. Being a melting down of the flesh and limbs into urine. Its cause is of a cold and humid nature as in dropsy. The course is the common one, namely, the kidneys and the bladder; for the patients never stop making water, but the flow is incessant, as if from the opening of aqueducts. The nature of the disease, then, is chronic, and it takes a long period to form; but the patient is short lived, if the constitution of the disease be completely established; for the melting is rapid, the death speedy. Moreover, life is disgusting and painful; thirst unquenchable; excessive drinking, which, however, is disproportionate to the large quantity of urine, for more urine is passed; and one cannot stop them either from drinking or making water; Or if for a time they abstain from drinking, their mouth becomes parched and their body dry; the viscera seem as if scorched up; they are affected with nausea, restlessness and a burning thirst...they stand out for a certain time, though not very long, for they pass urine with pain and the emaciation is dreadful; nor does any great portion of the drink get into the system, and many parts of the flesh pass out along with the urine.[3]

Aretaeus' writings were unknown in Europe until 1552. His aim in treating what was clearly type 1 diabetes was to overcome the intense thirst, and to this end he began with a purge and followed it with a variety of mixtures to soothe the stomach.

Galen (AD 129–210), whose teachings dominated Western medicine for more than a thousand years, mentions diabetes only briefly and regarded it as a kidney disease or, as he put it, 'diarrhoea of the urine'. He reported having seen only two sufferers, which, given that he had a large practice among the rich of Rome, seems odd. Perhaps most cases were among middle-aged epicureans whose symptoms were not striking? Physicians were expected to taste the urine to make a diagnosis, but screening those without symptoms in this way was perhaps beyond the call of duty. Galen's view that diabetes was a disease of the kidneys remained dominant in Europe throughout the Renaissance and lasted well into the nineteenth century.

The Persian physician and philosopher Avicenna (980–1037) was very familiar with diabetes, which he thought could be primary or secondary to another disease. He gave a comprehensive list of the symptoms and noted that, when the urine evaporated, it left a residue like honey. He also listed gangrene, carbuncles, and phthisis (tuberculosis) as complications.

The work of Avicenna and other Arab physicians and philosophers was not known in Europe, where the Church decreed that, since all knowledge was found in the Bible, there was no excuse for experiment. The revival of scientific medicine is often attributed to Theophastus Bombastus von Hohenheim (1493–1541), better known as Paracelsus, whose first public act when he became professor of medicine in Basel in 1526 was to burn the works of Galen and Avicenna. He ridiculed 'pisse prophets' who claimed to make diagnoses by inspecting the urine and suggested that the way forward was to analyse it chemically.

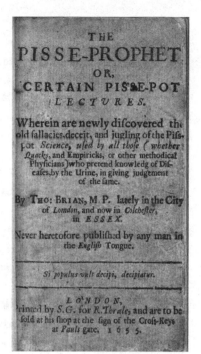

THE
PISSE-PROPHET
OR,
CERTAIN PISSE-POT
LECTURES.

Wherein are newly difcovered the
old fallacies, deceit, and jugling of the Pifs-
pot *Science, ufed by all thofe (whether
Quacks,* and Empiricks, or other methodical
Phyficians)who pretend knowledg of Dif-
eafes,by the Urine, in giving judgement
of the fame.

By THO: BRIAN, M.P. lately in the City
of *London,* and now in *Colcheſter,*
in *ESSEX.*

Never heretofore publifhed by any man in
the *Englifh* Tongue.

_____

Si populus vult decipi, decipiatur.

_____

LONDON,
Printed by S. G. for R. Thrale; and are to be
fold at his fhop at the fign of the Crofs-Keys
at *Pauls* gate, 1655.

2. Title page of a 1655 book ridiculing doctors who claimed to be able to make diagnoses by examining the urine. (*Wellcome Library, London*)

He evaporated the urine of a diabetic patient and obtained a white residue, which he mistook for salt. He thought diabetes was a tartaric disease (one of incrustation) due to a poisonous material (salt), which was deposited in the kidneys and bladder and stimulated them. Later he suggested that the seat of the disease was the stomach and the cause was blockage of the gastric veins by salt.

Given that tasting the urine was a relatively standard part of medical practice, it is surprising that the sweet taste of diabetic urine was apparently not known in Europe. One explanation is that diabetes was rare at a time when few were fat. Another is that it was only one cause of polyuria and that in the others, such as kidney failure, the urine was not sweet. Or it may have been noted but not publicized. In Europe the sweetness was 'discovered' by Thomas Willis (1621–75), who is remembered today for the description of the circle of arteries at the base of the brain that bears his name. His discourse on *Diabetes or the Pissing Evil* was published posthumously and in it he noted that 'diabetes was so rare among the ancients that many famous physicians did not mention it but in our age given to good fellowship and guzzling down of unallayed wine, we meet with examples and instances enough, I may say daily, of this disease'. He repeatedly writes of the urine as being 'exceedingly sweet' or 'wonderfully sweet like sugar or honey', but surprisingly did not consider that this might be because it contained sugar.[4]

That the sweetness was due to sugar was established by Matthew Dobson (1735–84), physician to the Liverpool Infirmary. In 1772 he admitted 33-year-old Peter Dickonson, who had had diabetic symptoms for eight months and was passing 28 pints (15 litres) of urine a day. He was emaciated and weak, with an unquenchable thirst. His urine was colourless, and Dobson evaporated 2 quarts, which left a white cake that could not 'by the taste be distinguished from sugar'. Dobson noted that the blood serum was 'sweetish' but not as sweet as the urine. He concluded that the kidneys excreted sugar that already existed in the blood, having been produced by fermentation in the stomach. Dickonson stayed in hospital for seven months and was given a variety of drugs, including rhubarb and senna (purgatives), Dover's powder (an opium-based mixture), and cantharides or Spanish Fly, a urinary irritant that was also used as an aphrodisiac. Eventually Dobson decided that his patient should drink the waters at Buxton spa in Derbyshire. He even provided expenses, but for some reason Dickonson never went. Maybe he had simply had enough of Dr Dobson's polypharmacy?

The Edinburgh physician William Cullen (1710–90) distinguished two forms of polyuria; that in which the urine was sweet he called *diabetes mellitus*, and when it was tasteless, *diabetes insipidus*, a name that is now used for the rare condition caused by deficiency of pituitary anti-diuretic hormone. In 1780 his colleague Francis Home (1719–1813), Professor of Materia Medica, treated two patients Arthur (aged 42) and Murray (24) and showed that diabetic urine could be fermented. He mixed half a pint of yeast with 24 pints of Arthur's urine: 'It soon began to ferment, and exit a vapour, like fermenting liquors. Next day it fermented strongly. On the third, the fermentation seemed over, it had lost all sweetness and tasted like small beer. Murray's treated in the same way, fermented into a tolerable small beer'.[5]

When Home tasted Arthur's and Murray's blood, neither seemed sweet, which, having read Dobson's paper, surprised him. He therefore concluded that sugar was made in the kidney or, if made in the gut, passed so quickly through the bloodstream that it could not be used. Apart from restriction of food, Arthur and Murray were given the usual cocktail of drugs: sudorifics (to promote sweating), anti-spasmodics, stimulants, tonics, astringents, and incrassants (to thicken the humours). Eventually Home concluded that his patients had tried all the treatments he had ever heard of. The older patient, Arthur, was discharged unchanged, while young Murray died.

Where the sugar in the urine came from was unclear, but an army surgeon John Rollo (d. 1809) thought it was formed in the stomach from vegetables. To him the obvious solution was to eliminate greens and to give a diet that consisted principally of animal food. The regimen published in his 1797 book *An Account of Two Cases of the Diabetes Mellitus* was:

First. The diet to consist of animal food principally, and to be thus regulated:

Breakfast. 1½ pints of milk and half a pint of lime water mixed together; bread and butter.

Lunch. Plain blood puddings, made of blood and suet only.

Dinner. Game or old meats which have been long kept; and as far as the stomach may bear, fat and rancid old meats, as pork. To eat in moderation.

Supper. The same as breakfast.

Secondly, a drachm of kali sulphuratum [potash] to be dissolved in four quarts of water which has been boiled, and to be used for daily drink. No other article whatever, either eatable or drinkable, to be allowed, than what has been stated.

Thirdly, the skin to be anointed with hog's lard every morning. Flannel to be worn next to the skin. The gentlest exercise only to be permitted: but confinement to be preferred.

Fourthly, a draught at bedtime of 20 drops of tartarized antimonial wine and 25 of tincture of opium; and the quantities to be gradually increased. In reserve as substances diminishing action, tobacco and foxglove (digitalis).

Fifthly, an ulceration about the size of a half crown to be produced and maintained externally, and immediately opposite to each kidney.

Sixthly, a pill of equal parts aloes and soap to keep the bowels regularly open.[6]

The diet gives just over 600 calories a day from carbohydrate and about 1,200 from fat. The ancillary treatments were standard for the time, and the only surprise is that bleeding, an almost universal treatment of any disease at the time, was not included.

The ulceration opposite each kidney was a method used in the eighteenth century to relieve congestion and inflammation of internal organs. Antimonial wine first surfaced in France in the seventeenth century as *vin émétique* and was promoted by William Cullen, under whom Rollo studied in Edinburgh. Rollo's first patient was an acquaintance, Captain Meredith of the Royal Artillery, whom Rollo had always thought a prime candidate for diabetes, as he was 'a large corpulent person'. After less than a month on the diet, Meredith was passing less urine and it no longer tasted sweet. This was a miracle to his servants, who tasted it out of curiosity! Meredith kept meticulous records of his urine volume and fluid intake, which he sent to Rollo. He lost nearly 50 lb (23 kg) in three months, and his daily urine volume fell from 12 litres to under 2. The second edition of Rollo's book in 1798 included another patient he had treated, a 'general officer', as well as communications from physicians who had written to him about their results with his treatment. During the last three months of his life the 57-year-old general returned to an unrestricted diet, including apple pudding and wine. This and experience with other patients led Rollo to lament:

> Our mode of treatment is so contrary to the inclinations of the sick. Though perfectly aware of the efficacy of the regimen, and the impropriety of deviations, yet they commonly trespass, concealing what they feel as a transgression on themselves. They express a regret that a medicine could not be discovered, however nauseous, or distasteful, which would supersede the necessity for any restriction in diet.

To the suggestion that Rollo's diet was unnatural, a London doctor insisted in 1862: 'This [living exclusively on meat] need not seem a mighty hardship: the iron-framed Esquimaux [Eskimos] do it, and the wiry, tough half-breds of the Pampas, with a bill of fare certainly less varied than our European meadows afford.'

The importance of Rollo's diet is that, albeit the premise was wrong, it was an attempt to treat diabetes rationally by preventing the formation of sugar. Until then treatment had involved giving a cocktail of drugs based on the old theory of humours. The obvious success of a meat (or low-carbohydrate) diet in getting rid of thirst and excessive urination made diet the preferred treatment of all physicians for the rest of the century.

Probably the only autobiographical account of diabetes and its treatment in the nineteenth century was published in 1858 by John Camplin, himself a doctor. He first had symptoms in 1844, when his colleagues predicted that treatment would only be 'smoothing my path to the grave'. At first he was advised to eat fat meat and eggs, but this produced 'great biliary derangement'. Later his advisers, who included two famous nineteenth-century doctors, William Prout (1785–1850) and Henry Bence Jones (1814–73), recommended:

> Meat, fish and eggs, with the cruciferae [cabbages and turnips]; they differed, however, in minor points; one advised coffee, another tea; one wine, and another brandy, &c; as a substitute for bread, cakes or biscuits made of washed flour and lard were at first recommended; these soon quite disagreed. The gluten bread was next tried; this latter, unpleasant as it was, I took as long as it could be borne.[7]

Later Prout introduced him to bran cake, which he described as 'by no means a pleasant composition but one which acted powerfully on the bowels'. This was desirable, since constipation was a major problem with diets that consisted of as much meat and fat as the patient could swallow (especially if they were also given opium, as most were), and it is no surprise that Rollo and his successors all prescribed generous amounts of purgatives such as rhubarb, aloes, colocynth, senna, magnesium sulphate, castor oil, and croton oil.

An important development during the nineteenth century was the invention of chemical methods of measuring the amount of sugar in the urine, so providing a better way of monitoring the success of treatment than tasting the urine. In 1815 the French chemist Eugene Chevreul (1786–1889) showed that the sugar in diabetic urine was glucose or grape sugar, and in the 1830s it was confirmed that the blood of diabetics also contained glucose. Karl August Trommer (1806–79) invented the first test for glucose in 1841. Urine was heated with blue cupric (copper) sulphate, and in the presence of a reducing substance such as glucose, red cuprous oxide was formed. The copper test was improved by Herrmann von Fehling (1812–85), and, although it was ideal for detecting glucose, ordinary doctors found it too complicated for measuring the amount of glucose, it was a useful test of the progress or otherwise of treatment. In 1862 William Roberts (1830–99) of Manchester described a method in which two samples of diabetic urine were put in flasks and a piece of yeast added to one. After twenty-four hours on a warm mantelpiece, glucose in the flask with yeast had fermented so that the specific gravity fell. The amount of glucose was equal to the difference of the specific gravity before and after fermentation × 0.23. This was promoted as ideal for the doctor who wanted to treat his cases of diabetes 'scientifically'. Its advantage was that everything necessary, except the urinometer for measuring specific gravity, could be found in an ordinary domestic kitchen. Measuring blood glucose was possible, but needed large volumes of blood, plenty of time and meticulous technique. It was hardly ever used in clinical practice until the development of micromethods after the First World War.

Being able to measure the amount of glucose in the urine enabled scientifically minded physicians to compare different diets. One of these was Frederick William Pavy (1829–1911), who spent his working life at Guy's Hospital investigating what he called 'one of the most inscrutable of diseases'. His colleague Sir William Gull asked satirically: 'What sin has Pavy committed or his fathers before him, that he should be condemned to spend his whole life seeking the cure of an incurable disease?'[8] In 1861 Pavy's patient Joseph North, aged 32, was in Guy's Hospital for four months on a variety of diets while Pavy tested his urine six times a day. The only thing that cleared glucose from his urine was, as Rollo had discovered half a century earlier, 'an animal diet' with little or no carbohydrate. Pavy regarded a lack of bread as the greatest privation and proposed three substitutes: gluten bread, invented in France, was 'like chewing india rubber'; the bran muffins favoured by Camplin were so hard as to be almost inedible, but, for those who could get them down, they led to a feeling of fullness. Pavy favoured his own invention—almond food. The basis of this was that almonds did not contain starch. They were ground to a fine powder and then made into a biscuit with flour and eggs.

One diet that had a short vogue in the 1850s was sugar feeding, brainchild of the well-known but eccentric French physician Pierre Piorry (1794–1879). He thought that diabetics lost weight and felt so weak because of the amount of sugar they lost in the urine and that replacing it should restore their strength. A house surgeon to the Leicester Infirmary reported three cases in the *British Medical Journal (BMJ)* in 1858. The patients, women aged 23, 25, and 14, were, in the language of the paper, 'ordered' to take ½ lb treacle each day. The first stuck it for four months, whereas the second refused after the third day and had honey instead. None got any benefit.

At the end of the nineteenth century several physicians championed 'cures' based on a specific dietary item. These included Donkin's skim-milk (1874), Mosse's potato (1902), and von Noorden's oatmeal cure (1903). They had in common periods of semi-starvation when the 'curative' item replaced food. For example, in the regimen of Arthur Scott Donkin of Sunderland, skim-milk was given at regular intervals and 'to the exclusion of other food for a longer or shorter period'. This was not to most patients' liking, and Donkin emphasized that it would work only if they were in 'isolated, special wards, and under the care of strictly trustworthy nurses'. Donkin noted sadly that, when his patients began to feel better, they indulged 'clandestinely in the most injurious of the prohibited articles of food'.[9]

The oatmeal cure was invented by the German Carl H. von Noorden (1858–1944), one of the most respected diabetes specialists at the beginning of the twentieth century. It consisted of several days of a carbohydrate-free diet, one or two vegetable days, and then a few oat days. William Osler used it, and in the 1909 edition of his textbook included the following recipe: '250 gm oatmeal, the same amount of butter and the whites of six or eight eggs constitute the day's food. The oatmeal is cooked for two hours, and the butter and albumin stirred in. It may be taken in four portions during the day. Coffee, tea, or whisky and water may be taken with it.'[10]

Osler gave no advice about what to do with the 6–8 egg yolks left over, but one commentator suggested that they could be used to make custard for the rest of the family. Some physicians proposed yet more drastic forms of dieting. In 1870, during the siege of Paris in the Franco-Prussian war, the French physician Apollinaire Bouchardat (1806–86) noticed that glucose disappeared from the urine in some of his patients as a result of starvation—all subsequent wars have been shown to be 'good for diabetes' in the sense that the incidence rates and mortality of type 2 fall. Bouchardat's advice to diabetics was 'mangez le moins possible'. This was carried a step further by the Italian-born physician Guglielmo Guelpa (1850–1930), who worked in Paris. In 1896 he showed that fasting and saline enemas made diabetics sugar free in three days. He attributed this to the elimination of waste products and toxins and claimed equally dramatic results in asthma, epilepsy, migraine, eczema, and various eye conditions. In 1910 he collated his experience in a book *Autointoxication et Désintoxication*, much of which was devoted to refuting his many critics. It would be easy to dismiss Guelpa as a crank, but autointoxication was taken very seriously in mainstream medicine. In 1913 a meeting on the topic at the Royal Society of Medicine in London lasted six evenings and involved sixty speakers; when the findings were published they covered 380 pages.

At this point it is pertinent to ask how effective dietary treatment was. The first problem, as Rollo had noticed at the end of the eighteenth century, was that many patients either could not, or would not, follow the diet. In the *BMJ* in 1865, a physician from East Anglia lamented that dieting 'may be comparatively easy to effect in private practice; but in the case of the poor, especially the outpatient poor, who cannot be made to understand the necessity of abstaining from bread, potatoes, apples etc., it becomes a very difficult task to teach them what to eat, drink and avoid'.[11]

Rollo's patients had longed for a drug, 'however nauseous', that would supersede dieting, and there were plenty on the market, although their use was disdained by experts, who believed that, if you gave a diabetic patient an inch, he would take a mile and abandon all pretence of diet. A US government publication in 1894 listed no less than forty-two anti-diabetic remedies including bromides, uranium nitrate, and arsenic. Apart from approved remedies there were the nostrums of the patent medicine men. The word 'patent' in this context is a misnomer, since to be patented the composition would have had to have been divulged. The British and American Medical Associations waged long campaigns against what they called secret remedies. In 1908 the *BMJ* published the compositions of popular diabetes and obesity cures. One was Vin Urane Pesqui, a small amount of uranium nitrate in old Bordeaux wine—uranium nitrate was widely used for diabetes and approved by mainstream physicians. According to the advertising blurb, it 'positively cures sugared diabetes, provided it is resorted to at an early stage and used during a sufficient length of time…as soon as the patient has made use of this wine, his thirst is allayed almost instantaneously; his strength reappears; all his functions are gradually restored'. Another nostrum was Dill's Diabetic Mixture, advertised as 'The only known remedy for this deadly disease. No dieting is necessary.' One-third of it was alcohol, a common feature of secret remedies and one that presumably made the patient feel better. A preparation called 'Expurgo Anti-Diabetes' was described by the *Journal of the American Medical Association (JAMA)* as such an evident nostrum that even intelligent laymen could not be deceived by it. Nevertheless, some medical journals had accepted adverts for it, and physicians of what *JAMA* described as 'a certain type' supplied testimonials that appeared prominently in the adverts. Later in the twentieth century such physicians would be called drug company whores.

For sufferers who could be persuaded to diet, the outcome depended critically on their age and whether they were thin or fat. Camplin noted that, 'where the disease attacked the thin and delicate', there was little hope. He told of 'a thin, delicate, young lady, highly nervous and excitable, whose sister had died of a similar disease', who, in spite of strictly adhering to a meat diet, sank rapidly into a coma. Before they died, the breath and urine of these young people had a curious smell, which was variously compared to chloroform, rotting apples, or hay. It was assumed to be the result of some sort of fermentation and also thought to cause the coma in which they eventually died. In 1857 the source of the smell was identified by a German doctor as acetone (nail varnish remover), and the ferric chloride and nitroprusside tests to detect it in the urine were introduced in 1865 and 1882 respectively. These gave advance warning that the patient was reaching the critical stage and might develop a coma at any time.

The classic description of diabetic coma is that of the German physician Adolf Kussmaul (1822–1902) in 1874. One of his patients was a 35-year-old woman who in 1869 first noted that her urine left white spots (of glucose) on her underclothes. (The equivalent sign in men was white spots on their highly polished shoes where urine had splashed on them.) In 1872 Kussmaul's patient had a raging thirst and became strikingly thin. Then one night:

> She awakened with great shortness of breath, complained
> of severe pains in the hypogastrium [upper abdomen] and

feeling very sick. Her condition rapidly became so disturb-
ing that the family physician asked me to come. I found her
lying in bed but in the greatest uneasiness, throwing herself
here and there and begging for help in the fear of death. She
seemed very pale, face and body cool, extremities cold, pulse
very small and fast, breathing loud, rapid and the respiratory movements strikingly large ... she sank soon afterwards
into a stuporous condition in which the great loud breathing
continued and died at nine o'clock at night.[12]

The most prominent feature of this condition was the contrast
between the general weakness and vigorous breathing, which
we still call Kussmaul respiration.

Most progress in unravelling the biochemistry of diabetic coma
was made by the German physician Bernard Naunyn (1839–1925)
and his pupils. The blood of patients with diabetic coma was
found to be acid, and in 1877 Naunyn's assistant poisoned rabbits
with hydrochloric acid, which produced deep laboured breathing with violent heaving of the chest. When he neutralized the
acid by injecting alkali, their condition was dramatically reversed;
one, which had been *in extremis*, jumped off the table! The similarity of the symptoms in acidotic rabbits and humans with diabetic
acidosis (Naunyn was the first to use this phrase and today we
usually talk about ketoacidosis) suggested that the human condition might be due to an acid generated in the body, and in 1884
this was identified as beta-hydroxybutyric acid, a breakdown
product of fat. Despite heroic measures such as purgation, alka-
line enemas, intravenous sodium bicarbonate, and injections of
strychnine and other stimulants, coma was incurable and the
cause of death in two-thirds of young diabetics.

From the middle of the nineteenth century many physicians believed that there were two distinct types of diabetes.

That which has just been described in young people with an acute onset and bad outcome the French physician Étienne Lancereaux (1829–1910) called *diabète maigre* (thin diabetes). By contrast, the diabetes of middle-aged overweight people, *diabète gras* (fat diabetes), came on gradually and was relatively indolent, so that sufferers could live with it for many years. Rollo's patient Captain Meredith, for example, survived for fifteen years. People with *diabète gras* did not fall into coma but were subject to complications affecting the eyes, kidneys, and nerves.

The ophthalmoscope, an instrument for looking at the back of the eye (the retina), had been invented in 1850, and by 1890 all the features of diabetic retinopathy had been described. The famous German ophthalmologist Julius Hirschberg (1843–1925) claimed that retinal changes could be found in most people who had had diabetes for ten years. He also proposed that diabetic retinopathy was specific and separate from albuminuric (hypertensive) retinopathy. After him opinion was divided; those who believed it was specific claimed the clinical picture was unique and could occur in diabetics without hypertension or albuminuria (protein in the urine). Others held that the changes were due to hardening of the arteries, that retinopathy did not correlate with the severity of diabetes (that is, its lethality), and was virtually confined to older patients with other vascular disease.

Nephritis or a problem with the kidney was regarded as part and parcel of diabetes in the nineteenth century. In 1801 the English physician Erasmus Darwin (1731–1802) recognized some diabetics whose urine could be coagulated by heat (which precipitates protein) and associated this with dropsy or general swelling. In 1848 Prout suggested that albuminuria was an ominous prognostic sign. In 1859 Wilhelm Griesinger (1817–68), better known as the founder of biological psychiatry, reported that half of sixty-four diabetic patients had kidney changes at autopsy, but, like all other writers until the 1930s, he attributed this to high blood pressure and atherosclerosis.

In England the expert on the clinical manifestations of diabetes was Pavy, who by 1894 claimed to have seen 2,642 cases in private practice. His 1862 book *On the Nature and Treatment of Diabetes* was the first English textbook on the disease. Pavy and other nineteenth-century physicians recognized impotence as a common symptom, often the presenting one. Pavy described it in typically circumlocutory language: 'What has been said in respect of muscular action will apply also in explanation of the loss of virility which accompanies the inveterate form of the disease. The condition which the blood presents may be considered as unsuited for the maintenance of functional activity in the organs in question.'[13] A description of diabetic nerve damage, which would not be out of place in a modern textbook, was given by Pavy in 1885. He wrote:

> The usual account given by these patients of their condition is that they cannot feel properly in their legs, that their feet are numb, that their legs seem too heavy—as one patient expressed it, 'as if he had 20 lb weights on his legs and a feeling as if his boots were a great deal too large for his feet'. Darting or 'lightning' pains are often complained of. Or there may be hyperaesthesia, so that a mere pinching of the skin gives rise to great pain; or it may be the patient is unable to bear the contact of the seam of the dress against the skin on account of the suffering it causes. Not infrequently there is deep-seated pain, located, as the patient describes it, in the marrow of the bones which are tender on being grasped, and I have noticed that these pains are generally worse at night.[14]

As treatment, Pavy recommended opium or codeine and, if this did not work, 'continuous galvanic current'. Where the main symptom was superficial pain, he suggested 'cautious application of the linimentum aconiti' (an alkaloid from the monk's hood plant). Their modern equivalents are transcutaneous electrical nerve stimulation (TENS) and capsaicin cream.

Pavy pointed out that neuropathy made the feet of the diabetic extremely vulnerable, so that 'a very trivial injury may suffice to lead to the establishment of serious mischief, involving often a more or less extensive loss of living parts and, it may be, even the loss of life'. The particular mischief he was referring to was the perforating ulcer, about which he wrote:

> A spot of surface mischief becomes perceptible and remains without exhibiting any sign of healing action. An incrustation may form under which ulceration may proceed and by-and-by a burrowing sinus may be discovered leading, it may be, into the joint of a toe or to denuded bone. Sometimes this condition is attended with such little surface appearance as to lead to surprise being experienced when the extent to which deep-seated mischief has advanced is discovered. Sometimes the mischief remains restricted to the surface. The part simply fails to possess the requisite healing power to become reinstated and the sore persists in an indolent state. There is usually a prolonged history of peripheral neuritis.[15]

Ulcers and gangrene of the feet were not uncommon, but, before the introduction of antisepsis by Lister in 1865, conventional teaching had been not to amputate for diabetic gangrene because of a near certainty that the stump would not heal and the gangrene would spread. With antisepsis, the risk of infection was to some extent reduced, but surgeons invariably recommended amputation above the knee and would continue to do so well into the twentieth century to be sure that the wound would heal.

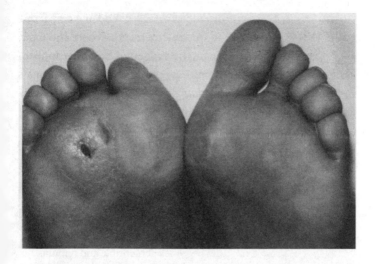

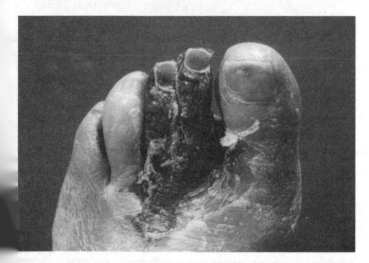

3. The two main types of diabetic foot problem. At the top is a perforating ulcer due to neuropathy. Below are the gangrenous second and third toes due to blocked arteries.

Apart from amputations, the only other time Victorian surgeons were involved was in the treatment of carbuncles, which are basically large boils, most commonly on the back of the neck. In the pre-antibiotic days they were particularly common with diabetes, because high blood glucose levels interfere with some of the body's defences against bacterial infection. Carbuncles could be as large as grapefruits or melons, but, although treated by excision or cauterization, were often fatal, because the bacteria spread to the bloodstream, causing septicaemia.

II

UNRAVELLING THE ROLE
OF THE PANCREAS

I n the early nineteenth century the standard way of finding out which organ was involved with a group of symptoms was opening the body after death. Thus most people who had wasted away and coughed up blood were found to have characteristic lesions in the lungs—the tubercles of phthisis or pulmonary tuberculosis. In this condition, using a stethoscope or percussing the chest with the fingers could predict the presence of cavities or consolidation in the lung in life. Another striking example of the value of correlating clinical and autopsy findings was the work of Thomas Addison of Guy's Hospital, London, who in 1855 described a disease in which the sufferers became very tired and had a peculiar darkening of the skin. His first five patients with what became known as Addison's disease all had changes in the adrenal glands, which had previously been thought to be vestigial structures.

Where diabetes was concerned, autopsies were unhelpful. In spite of the excessive urination, the kidneys looked normal, as did all other organs to the naked eye. Because knowledge of its cause was so sketchy, textbook writers had difficulty in knowing in which section to put diabetes. In the first edition of his textbook in 1892, Osler included it with gout under 'constitutional diseases'. Others still put it in the section on kidney diseases, and in a 1901 book it was described as 'a "general disease" which has no local seat, which is certainly not a disease of the kidney...We therefore place it by itself as a non-febrile general disease, with no ascertained pathology or anatomy.'[1]

Irrespective of which organ was involved, physicians in the first half of the nineteenth century had little doubt that 'grief', 'chills', and 'an excess of venery' were contributory factors. John Elliotson (1791–1868), later sacked from University College for supporting Mesmerism, was puzzled by a patient who died of diabetes but claimed he had never known a woman. Elliotson thought it 'very possible that he had committed excess of a less creditable kind', the evidence being that he had an abnormally long prepuce. Prout implicated 'the noxious weed' tobacco.[2]

Also, as had been noted by Indian physicians 1,000 years earlier, diabetes ran in families. Up to a quarter of sufferers knew of an affected relative, and there were many reports of families with multiple diabetic members. A striking case was described by Pavy in which a man sired sons by three different women and all later developed diabetes. Following the discovery of the bacterial origin of many diseases in the 1880s, it was natural to wonder whether diabetes might be contagious. At a meeting in 1896 a French doctor presented some remarkable histories that supported the idea; a laundress became diabetic after washing the linen of a man and his little daughter, who both had the disease; in another the mother became diabetic, then her son, next the cook who had washed handkerchiefs for her master, and lastly a sewing woman who used to go to the house. Another possible example of infectious diabetes was the situation where both husband and wife were affected.

A major conceptual breakthrough came from Claude Bernard (1813–78), one of the greatest physiologists of the nineteenth century and founder of experimental medicine. When he began his work in 1843, received wisdom was that only plants could make sugar and that animal metabolism consisted in breaking down substances originally made in plants. It was also thought that the blood of animals contained sugar only after meals or in pathological states such as diabetes. Between 1846 and 1848 Bernard found that sugar was present in the blood of normal animals, even when starved, which at first he found so astonishing that he doubted his analytical method. He also found a higher concentration of sugar in the hepatic vein, which leads from the liver to the general circulation, than in the portal vein, which takes blood from the intestine to the liver. Hence, he surmised, the liver must be secreting sugar, and in the liver he found a large amount of a starch-like substance, which we now know is composed of glucose molecules. He called this glycogen (sugar forming) and compared it to starch in plants. The crucial experiment was that, when he took a slice of liver immediately after the death of an animal and put it in boiling water, he got an opalescent liquid that tested negative for sugar. However, if he added saliva (which contains enzymes that break down glycogen), the liquid cleared and the test for sugar became strongly positive. His hypothesis, the glycogenic theory, was that sugar absorbed from the intestine was converted into glycogen in the liver and then constantly released into the blood during fasting.

Bernard's fame was so great that young physicians clamoured to work with him. In 1852, one such was Frederick Pavy, who spent the rest of his life trying to disprove the glycogenic theory. He thought Bernard, whom he always called 'this celebrated physiologist', had been misled into inferring a physiological condition from post-mortem findings. In life, Pavy insisted, there was only a trace of sugar in the blood between the liver and lungs—methods of measuring blood sugar were so complex that it was difficult to prove this one way or the other. Far from making sugar, Pavy insisted, the liver was a barrier preventing sugar reaching the general circulation, whence it would have been lost in the urine. He believed (wrongly) that the kidney was a simple filter, so that, if any glucose was present in the blood, it would pass into the urine. Bernard maintained (correctly) that the kidney was a dam that held back sugar until the level in the blood exceeded 11 mmol/l (200 mg/dl). This became known as the renal threshold for glucose, and we now know that it varies from person to person. The main premise for Pavy's objection to the glycogenic theory was the natural theology argument that nature would behave in a common-sense way and that changing sugar into glycogen and back again was 'not what we should expect from the notion we possess of the manner in which the operations of nature are conducted'. In fact, although Pavy did not know it, the brain needs a constant supply of glucose from the blood, and, without glycogen, life would be impossible.

Another English physician who studied with Bernard was George Harley (1829–96), who aspired to be a scientific physician, unlike most of his colleagues, who had no interest in research. He would probably have become as or more influential than Pavy in England had it not been for an eye disease that forced him to abandon experimental medicine. He totally accepted the glycogenic theory and thought it obvious that animals must be able to synthesize sugars. Bernard had shown that dogs fed an exclusively meat diet had sugar in their blood, and 'where', asked Harley, 'does the sugar in a polar bear's milk come from if it is not manufactured by some organ in the animal's own body?'[3]

Bernard's research suggested that the liver was one organ involved in diabetes. Harley, who had suggested in 1866 that there were two types of diabetes, believed that in what he called 'fat and ruddy' patients the cause was overproduction of sugar by the liver. Pavy was sceptical but did record the case of a man who developed diabetes after being kicked over the liver by a horse.

Another organ that was thought to be involved was the brain. Prout had noted (wrongly) that animals did not get diabetes and asked, 'Can the exception be referred to that fertile cause of bodily disorder in human beings, the influence of the mind?'[4] However, it was almost certainly Bernard's *piqûre* experiment in 1849 that focused attention on the brain. This discovery came about because Bernard had found that cutting the vagus nerve abolished the secretion of glucose by the liver. He tried the process in reverse by stimulating the vagus, but found no effect. He therefore decided to prick the point in the fourth ventricle of the brain where the vagus arises and 'I succeeded at the first attempt in making the animal diabetic. At the end of an hour, the blood and urine of the animal were full of sugar.' This effect lasted only as long as glycogen remained in the liver. If the animal had been starved to exhaust liver glycogen, there was no glycosuria (glucose in the urine). The fact that *piqûre* diabetes was always temporary seems to have been ignored, and between 1860 and 1900 the nervous origin of diabetes was much discussed. Facts that were alleged to support it were cases that started soon after a nervous shock and, according to Robert Saundby, 'the well known fact that the disease is much more common among the educated than the uneducated classes—that is it occurs chiefly among those whose nervous systems undergo more wear and tear'.[5] It was also said that diabetes was more common among engine drivers than other railway workers because of the arduous nature of their work— the possibility that firemen were protected by their much more physical job was not considered.

It was diabetes in older fatter people that was thought to be connected with the liver and/or nervous system. The cause of the disease in thin young people was a total mystery until the announcement by Oskar Minkowski (1858–1931), at the International Congress of Physiology in September 1889, that removal of the pancreas in dogs caused severe diabetes. The function of the pancreas had been totally unknown until 1848, when Claude Bernard established that it produced digestive enzymes. There had been occasional reports of pancreatic disease and diabetes in the same person, but this was regarded as coincidental, because Bernard had tied the pancreatic ducts of animals without producing diabetes in spite of the fact that the pancreas had almost withered away.

Minkowski was born in Kaunas (now in Lithuania). After qualifying as a doctor in 1881, he worked in Königsberg with Bernhard Naunyn and moved with him to Strassburg (now Strasbourg) in 1888. There he and Josef von Mering (1849–1908) discussed the function of the pancreas. Minkowski suggested that the way to find out what it did was to remove it, and, since a spare dog was available, they went ahead that afternoon. What drew Minkowski's attention to diabetes was that, some days after the operation, the lab man told him that the previously house-trained dog was urinating everywhere. Minkowski criticized him for not letting it out often enough, to which the lab man replied that letting it out made no difference. This prompted Minkowski to test the urine, which was loaded with sugar. The illness of the dog without a pancreas was very similar to that of humans with *diabète maigre*.

Minkowski admitted that his discovery was a lucky accident, but other circumstances were propitious. He was working in a department where diabetes was the main subject of study and experimental work was encouraged; it was also before the days of ethics committees! His surgical ability made the discovery possible, and he understood the implications from the beginning and followed it up over many years.

The announcement that pancreatectomy caused diabetes was a surprise but was soon confirmed in France and Germany. Possible explanations were that the pancreas might

1. destroy sugar coming to it in the blood;
2. produce an enzyme that destroyed sugar in the blood;
3. destroy a toxin made elsewhere in the body that interfered with sugar metabolism;
4. produce an internal secretion (later called a hormone).

Transplantation experiments were the most convincing evidence for the internal secretion theory. Minkowski cut the pancreas of a dog in half and transplanted one half into the abdominal wall, where it took root. When he removed the half left in the abdomen, diabetes did not develop. However, when the abdominal wall transplant was removed, the animals became diabetic. The French physiologists Edouard Hédon (1863–1933) and Jules Thiroloix (1861–1932) did similar experiments, as did Gustave Laguesse (1861–1927), who suggested that the putative internal secretion was produced by the 'small irregularly polygonal cells, with brilliant cytoplasm, diffusely scattered in the pancreatic parenchyma', which had been discovered in 1869 by Paul

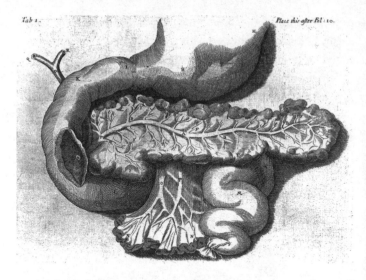

4. 1676 drawing of the pancreas with its head, as my anatomy teachers said, 'nestling in the arms of the duodenum'. (*Wellcome Library, London*)

Langerhans (1847–88), as a medical student in Berlin.[6] These are still called the islets or islands of Langerhans.

The originator of the internal-secretion theory was Charles-Édouard Brown-Séquard (1817–93), one of the most colourful scientists of the nineteenth century. Born in Mauritius of an American sea captain and a French mother, he moved to Paris aged 20. He had a flair for self-publicity, and one series of experiments that brought him early notoriety was on the mechanism of rigor mortis, for which he used the bodies of guillotined criminals into which he transfused blood (often his own). He was well known in England, where in 1860 he became a founding physician at the National Hospital, Queen Square. In London he became a victim of his own success, and it is said that he decided to leave when he looked out of his consulting-room window and saw the square outside gridlocked by the carriages of his fashionable patients. He was an extraordinarily energetic man, who often worked 20 hours a day and published 577 papers during his career. He crossed the Atlantic more than sixty times and set up residence in America four times, France six times, England once, and Mauritius twice.

In 1869, during research on the adrenal gland, Brown-Séquard had suggested that all glands with (exocrine) or without ducts (endocrine) 'supplied to the blood substances which are useful or essential and the lack of which may produce physiological signs'. In June 1889, three months before Minkowski's presentation, he gave a lecture that, in the words of the *BMJ*, 'caused the idea of internal secretion to take possession of the general imagination'. At the Société de Biologie in Paris the septuagenarian described how he had prepared testicular fluid from animals and injected himself with it every day for two weeks. As a result, he claimed to have been rejuvenated. The evidence was that he was much more vigorous, could lift heavy weights, and could run upstairs. Also the average length of his jet of urine had increased by 25 per cent. English doctors wrote to the *BMJ* complaining that the experiments were disgusting and unnatural. This was partly because Brown-Séquard had suggested that masturbation without ejaculation might have the same effect. One correspondent wrote that 'vivisection may be an open question but self-abuse is not!' Since Brown-Séquard was well known in England and America, his views, although greeted with some scepticism and lampooned by cartoonists, were taken seriously, and in 1893 the *BMJ* published two of his papers in which he stated that there was no doubt that the pancreas had an internal secretion that was even more important

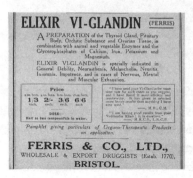

5 An advertisement for an organotherapy panacea, *Medical
Annual*, 1900.

than its external one. He recommended the simultaneous use
of orchitic (testicular) and pancreatic liquid in all cases of diabetes. Immodestly he concluded that 'the great movement in
therapeutics as regards the organic liquid extracts has origin in
the experiments I made on myself in 1889, experiments which
were at first so completely misunderstood'.[7] In an accompany-
ing editorial the *BMJ* worried that there might be 'an epidemic
of universal injections',[8] and this was exactly what happened.
The pharmaceutical industry was quick to exploit the organotherapy craze that Brown-Séquard had started. Extracts of
many organs were commonly combined, as shown in Fig. 5, the
justification being that the body would take what it needed and
reject the rest.

In an address to the annual meeting of the British Medical
Association in 1895 the physiologist Edward Schäfer (1850–1935)
endorsed Brown-Séquard's view that many organs produced
an internal secretion and concluded that the subject had a vast
future. In relation to diabetes he wrote:

> The only fact that appears certain in connection with the
> manner in which the pancreas prevents excessive production
> of sugar within the body is that this effect must be produced

by the formation of some material, secreted internally by the gland and probably by the internal vascular islets, and that the internally secreted material profoundly modifies the carbohydrate metabolism of the tissues.[9]

The English physiologist Ernest Starling (1866–1927) first used the name 'hormone' in 1905. It comes from the Greek word meaning to stir up, and it soon came to be applied, in Starling's words, to 'any substance normally produced in the cells of one part of the body and carried by the bloodstream to distant parts, which it affects for the good of the organism as a whole'.[10]

One powerful piece of evidence for internal secretions was the dramatic effects of thyroid extract. At a meeting in Durham in 1891, George Redmayne Murray (1865–1939) presented a 46-year-old woman with florid underactivity of the thyroid gland (myxoedema) and described how he intended to treat her with sheep thyroid extract. On twice-weekly injections she gradually improved and within six months was cured, albeit she had to keep taking the medicine to stay well. It was soon shown that thyroid extract was equally effective by mouth, and this led to attempts to cure diabetes by pancreas feeding. These trials were done without any clear end points, except whether the patients felt better and had less sugar in their urine, and all were failures. In fact, the apparent normality of the pancreas at autopsy led many to deny the connection of the pancreas with diabetes. Many physicians found it difficult to imagine that the islets of Langerhans, comprising only 1 per cent of the pancreas, could be responsible for controlling carbohydrate metabolism. Changes in the islets under a microscope had been noted, although this work was not widely known or appreciated. In 1899 Leonid V. Sobolev (1876–1919) suggested that the islets were functionally and

anatomically independent of the rest of the pancreas and controlled carbohydrate metabolism. In four out of fifteen cases
of diabetes he found that islets had totally disappeared, while
in nine there were fewer than normal. Presciently he suggested
that 'by ligating the pancreatic duct we now have a means of
isolating the islands anatomically and of studying their chemical products freed from the digestive ferments. This anatomic
isolation will permit the testing, in a rational way, of an organotherapy for diabetes.'[11]

Like Sobolev, the American Eugene Opie (1873–1971) thought
the islets were secretory organs rather than modified exocrine
cells. He suggested that severe damage to them resulted in diabetes, and this was supported by finding hyalinized (obliterated)
islets in autopsies of juvenile diabetics.

Between 1900 and 1921 at least five investigators came close to
discovering the hypothetical islet hormone, which the Belgian
Jean de Meyer had named 'insuline' in 1909.

At a meeting in Paris in 1922 Eugène Gley (1857–1930) asked
that an envelope deposited by him in 1905 be opened. In it he
described how he had tied off the pancreatic ducts in animals
and, when the pancreas had withered, prepared extracts of what
was left. When injected, they decreased the glycosuria of depancreatized dogs and alleviated their symptoms. Why he did not
pursue his ideas is unknown.

In 1903 John Rennie (1865–1928), a zoologist, and Thomas
Fraser (1872–1951), a physician in Aberdeen, Scotland made
extracts of islets of cod and hake, which, unlike those of mammals, are separate from the exocrine pancreas. Five patients
were treated by mouth without success. In 1904 they gave the
extract to another patient by hypodermic injection daily for
six days but gave up because of side effects. Urine volume and

glycosuria were unaffected, and they concluded either that they had not given enough extract or that a fish product would not work in mammals. (Fish insulin does work in man and was used in Japan during the Second World War when other types were not available.)

In 1906, in Berlin, Georg Zuelzer (1870–1949) tied the pancreatic ducts of animals and, after the organ had shrivelled, squeezed out the juice, precipitated the proteins with alcohol, and injected the extract. He treated eight patients and concluded that glycosuria and ketonuria (acetone or ketones in the urine) could be eliminated without any change in diet. His extract was tested in Minkowski's unit on three dogs and three patients, but, although he was able to confirm that it suppressed glycosuria, the side effects were so severe that it was thought to be unsafe. After the discovery of insulin, Minkowski blamed himself for not investigating the side effects more thoroughly, since the drug obviously worked. Zuelzer continued his experiments and in 1913 persuaded the drug company Hoffman La Roche to make an extract, which was abandoned when it produced severe convulsions—almost certainly due to low blood sugar (hypoglycaemia).

Another who might have succeeded was Ernest Scott (1877–1966), who in 1908 went to the University of Chicago to work with the newly appointed Professor of Physiology, Anton J. Carlson. Rather than tying off the duct, Scott extracted fresh pancreas with alcohol. His extract produced a significant drop in urinary glucose in three of four dogs. The conclusions he drew in his thesis submitted to the University of Chicago in 1911 were that:

> 1st, there is an internal secretion from the pancreas controlling the sugar metabolism.

2nd, by proper methods this secretion may be extracted and still retain its activity.

3rd, this secretion is easily destroyed by oxidation or by the action of the digestive enzymes of the pancreas.[12]

Unfortunately, by the time Scott's paper was published, a sentence had been inserted warning: 'It does not follow that these effects are due to the internal secretion of the pancreas in the extract.' Scott's wife believed that what she called that damning sentence had been introduced by Carlson, whom she described pejoratively as 'a recent Swedish immigrant' compared to her husband, 'a fourth generation Ohio farm boy'. After moving to Kansas, Scott maintained his interest in the pancreas and in 1912 visited the physiologist J. J. R. Macleod, who was working in Cleveland, Ohio. According to Scott, Macleod was not interested and 'just shrugged it off'. This is not surprising, because in 1921, in his highly successful textbook of physiology, Macleod wrote:

The removal of some hormone necessary for proper sugar metabolism is, however, by no means the only way in which the results [of pancreatectomy] can be explained, for we can assume that the pancreas owes its influence over sugar metabolism to some change occurring in the composition of the blood as this circulates through the gland—a change which is dependent on the integrity of the gland and not on any one enzyme or hormone which it produces.[13]

Scott later attributed his failure to not measuring blood sugar—his method needed 20cc for each measurement and would have exsanguinated even relatively large animals during a thirty-six-hour experiment.

In 1919, at the Rockefeller Institute in New York, Israel Kleiner (1885–1966) tested a pancreatic extract intravenously in sixteen depancreatized dogs and found a substantial reduction of blood sugar in most. Kleiner thought the temporary effect might be useful in emergencies in man. He also noted that it was simple to make and did not have any toxic effects, although he did worry that animal extracts would not work in humans. Others do not appear to have shared this concern, presumably because animal thyroid extracts worked in man.

The failure to isolate an effective pancreatic extract and the fact that the pancreas appeared normal at autopsy led many to doubt the relevance of the pancreas to most cases of human diabetes, for which the number of potential causes was immense. In 1912 the English physician Archibald Garrod, famous for having discovered the inherited diseases called inborn errors of metabolism, gave a series of lectures at the Royal College of Physicians. He regarded it as well established that diabetes was a syndrome, but the causes included 'a medley of conditions, many of which stand in no obvious relationship to each other'.[14] Garrod's list ranged from poisons such as atropine, curare, and strychnine through anaesthetics to alcohol—especially, according to him, that in champagne and beer. It also included asphyxia, psychic shock, diseases of the nervous system, liver, and pancreas, and diseases of the thyroid and pituitary glands. Other less scientific doctors simply blamed lifestyle. In the same year as Garrod's lecture a Canadian doctor suggested:

> The majority of patients suffer from the disease because they have ignorantly or carelessly abused their systems with the amount or the kind of food they have eaten or by their method of eating. Improper insalivation of the food, due to the pernicious habit of 'bolting' it, too large an amount, mental concentration such as thinking deeply, reading or worrying while eating, all tend to produce that disarrangement of metabolism which exhibits itself as diabetes.[15]

Failure to chew food adequately was widely regarded as unhealthy, and the movement that recommended thorough chewing was called Fletcherism.

The Canadian's formulation did have the merit of suggesting a method of prevention and—namely, eating less and worrying less—and many doctors promoted these. In the 1909 edition of his best-selling textbook, Osler recommended: 'Sources of worry should be avoided, and [the diabetic patient] should lead an even quiet life, if possible in an equable climate.'[16] The rest of his prescription is devoted to the principles of a low-carbohydrate diet. Osler explicitly states that he is talking about *diabète gras* and indicates that the outlook for *diabète maigre* was hopeless. It was, since 90 per cent of those who developed diabetes under the age of 20 died within two years.

The person who did most to alter this bleak outlook was an American doctor, Frederick Madison Allen (1876–1964). Between 1909 and 1912 he did three years' intensive research on diabetes at Harvard, but, because his papers were so long, no journal would publish them. So he borrowed $5,000 from his father to print *Studies Concerning Glycosuria and Diabetes* (1913), a tome of 1,179 pages in which he produced an exhaustive review of the literature on metabolism in general and diabetes in particular. Allen did animal experiments in which he removed varying amounts of the pancreas to produce the equivalents of severe or mild human diabetes—what we would call types 1 and 2. Dogs left with 20 per cent of their pancreas or more did not develop diabetes. The fate of those with 80–90 per cent of their pancreas removed depended on what they ate. If fed a low-carbohydrate diet, they remained relatively well, like middle-aged humans with diabetes—since Eskimos lived on 52 grams of carbohydrate daily, Allen called this an Eskimo diet. Large amounts of carbohydrate (which Allen called a Hindu diet) wore out the pancreatic remnant, and what had originally been mild diabetes turned into the severe form. From this Allen decreed that patients should order their lives 'according to the size of their pancreas'. Basically this meant reducing food intake until the urine was sugar free. In 1914 he was given a junior position at the Rockefeller Institute in New York, where there was no shortage of clients, since physicians were only too willing to send him their 'hopeless' diabetics. His first findings on forty-four patients were published in 1915 under the title 'Prolonged fasting in diabetes'. This article was picked up by the *Daily Mail*, which announced that a cure for diabetes had been found—such hyperbolic headlines continue in the twenty-first century as shown below.

> Diabetes is ancient and anything but mild (*The Times*, 18 Nov. 1999, 44).
>
> Twice-yearly diabetic jab (*Daily Mail*, 4 Apr. 2000, 9).
>
> Diabetes defeated in 10 years (*Scotsman*, 27 Jan. 2001, 1).
>
> Diabetes devours NHS billions as Britain gets fatter (*Sunday Times*, 17 Mar. 2001, 8).
>
> Diabetes set to swallow a fifth of NHS budget by 2010 (*Sunday Telegraph*, 10 June 2001, 6).
>
> Cod liver oil may prevent diabetes (*Daily Telegraph*, 2 Nov. 2001, 5).
>
> Drinkable insulin breakthrough (*Scotsman*, 29 Apr. 2002, 1).
>
> Pain-free insulin patch for diabetes (*Guardian*, 9 Apr. 2004, 6).
>
> 40-minute op to beat diabetes (*Daily Mail*, 5 June 2007, 44).
>
> Diabetes drug that could cut deaths by 40 per cent (*Mail on Sunday*, 31 Mar. 2008, 41).

Editorialists in the *Lancet* and *BMJ* were extremely critical of the *Daily Mail* in particular, and sensationalist newspapers in general. Neither were they impressed by Allen's paper, which the *Lancet* damned with faint praise, saying 'we are inclined to think that the discomfort which it [fasting] entails will seriously militate against its general use, even if further experience substantiates its merit'.[17] In 1919 Allen wrote *Total Dietary Regulation in the Treatment of Diabetes*, a volume of 646 pages plus charts. He was an unattractive person, described as a 'square-faced stern-looking man who never smiled and who attempted to exercise control over his patients like his laboratory animals'.[18] The initial diet he put his patients on for ten days was:

> Water 1,500–2,000 cc per day.
> Coffee 1–3 cups.
> Clear meat soup, up to 600 cc.
>
> Bran muffins 3–6 (to produce satiety and combat constipation).

When the urine was sugar free, carbohydrate tolerance was determined by adding increasing amounts of vegetables until sugar reappeared. Protein was then added and finally fat, until the calorific value of the diet was 'sufficient'. The daily average energy intake was 1,956 calories, of which 8 per cent was carbohydrate, 22 per cent protein, and 70 per cent fat. To put this into context, nutritionists at the time advised that a 3,000-calorie diet for a working man should obtain 66 per cent of calories from carbohydrate, 16 per cent from protein, and 18 per cent from fat. The novel aspect of Allen's treatment was his insistence that severe diabetics should be kept permanently underweight. The previous philosophy had been that, after fasting had abolished glycosuria, patients should be fattened up and strengthened by the addition of as many non-carbohydrate calories as possible.

A similar diet was devised at St Bartholomew's Hospital, London, by George Graham (1882–1971), like Allen an austere and humourless bachelor. The main difference was that, whereas Allen's patients were active and went out to concerts, Graham's stayed in bed, so the ward sister could keep a careful watch on them. They still managed to get carbohydrate surreptitiously, but Graham justified bed rest because, 'if the diabetic learns to lie still in bed, he will have a much lower basal metabolism and therefore will be able to live in comparative comfort on a low caloric diet'.[19]

Starvation treatment did work in a limited sense and was welcomed by some doctors simply because they had nothing else to offer. One of its most enthusiastic proponents was Elliott Joslin (1869–1962), who became the most famous diabetes specialist of the twentieth century. The first edition of his textbook *The Treatment of Diabetes Mellitus* was published in 1916, and for it he managed to trace 97.5 per cent of the thousand patients he had seen during the previous twenty years. Joslin was paternalistic and puritan, but these traits were tempered by charm, warmth, and optimism, and his patients loved him. He was probably one of the first doctors in the twentieth century who not only preached the importance of patient education but also practised it. He eulogized what he called the simplicity of Allen's under-nutrition treatment, because it delivered the patient 'from medicines, patent and otherwise, sham kinds of treatment [and] gluten breads'.[20] Another enthusiast was the German-born Otto Leyton (1873–1938) of the London Hospital, who warned that 'patients below a certain standard of intellect, and possessing no self control, cannot be treated because they are unable to grasp the gravity of the disease from which they are suffering, and to adhere to the diet when free from control'.[21]

Leyton wrote that the doctor needed to persuade the patient to look on him as a friend not a jailer, but his language suggests the exact opposite. For example, if the patient was in a nursing home, it should be one where 'the matron has sufficient control over every department to be certain that orders are carried out'. Leyton's patients were initially forgiven the *first act of disobedience*, but later were sent home for *the first offence*.

Character was a crucial factor in the success or otherwise of under-nutrition treatment. In 1921 John R. Williams of New York claimed that most failures were due to 'unfaithfulness on the part of the patient' and nearly half the deaths in his seventy-three patients were because the treatment had been abandoned. His harsh comment was that 'many cases unquestionably die because of lack of courage'.[22] Allen also talked about 'the habitually unfaithful type of patient', but was sufficiently astute to point out that 'fidelity' (which would now be called compliance) could not be predicted from intelligence or social position. Allen also claimed that many patients died because 'ignorant' doctors did not understand his regimen.

Unfortunately for many *faithful* patients, the result was literal starvation and some died of inanition, not diabetes. In 1921 the most famous European diabetes specialist, Carl von Noorden, turned away in disapproval when he saw Joslin's prize patient, 17-year-old Ruth A., who at just over 5 feet weighed only 54 lb (24.5 kg). Rawle Geyelin (1883–1942) of New York gave numbing descriptions of the pitiful state of such patients in a 1923 paper. A 15-year-old girl who had had diabetes for three years weighed 46¾ lb and went home on 6 grams of carbohydrate, 25 grams of protein, and 30 grams of fat per day. A 10-year-old boy who had had diabetes for 4½ years weighed only 27 lb (12.3 kg) and was so weak he could not lift his head from the pillow.

At a meeting in 1921 most London teaching-hospital consultants were enthusiastic about the fasting treatment; one dissenter was Frederick Poynton of Great Ormond Street Hospital, who described the disappointing results in children. Later he published the cases of five who all died within thirty months. In each case the parents went through three stages:

> First, the thought that they were succeeding, then the uneasy feeling that they were losing, and finally the realisation that we protracted the illnesses, but nothing more, and the very partial success was so unsatisfactory from the children's point of view that, had not there always been a hope that some new advance might appear, or some unexpected improvement arise, it hardly seemed worthwhile.[23]

In a 1922 lecture Joslin posed the rhetorical question: 'Since diabetes is always fatal in children, why prolong the agony? Why not let the poor child eat and be happy while life lasts?' His answer was that 'no man knows but that the cure may be at hand within the year—even the month'. In fact, he did know about the dramatic discovery described in the next chapter.

III

⠦

INSULIN:
A force of magical activity

After the horrors of the First World War, the early 1920s were, as the historian E. H. Carr said, a time for 'reconstruction, restoration and recovery'. A striking symbol of this new optimism was the long-awaited isolation of the internal secretion of the pancreas, described in a letter to *The Times* as 'a force of magical activity'.

The story of how insulin was discovered in Toronto in 1921 is well known, at least in a simplified outline. A young orthopaedic surgeon, Frederick Banting, reads an article on diabetes and has the idea that others have missed the anti-diabetic principle of the pancreas because it was digested by enzymes during the extraction process. He will overcome this by tying the pancreatic duct so that the enzyme-producing part of the pancreas degenerates. He approaches J. J. R. Macleod, now working in Toronto, who, as he had done with Scott (see Chapter 2), pours scorn on the idea. Eventually Macleod relents, loans him a lab, and goes on holiday to Scotland. A student, Charles Best, is chosen to help Banting, and within six months they make one of the most important medical discoveries ever. All turns sour when the 1923 Nobel Prize is awarded jointly to Banting and Macleod.

Banting is so angry that he announces publicly that he will share his prize with Best, whereupon Macleod does the same with Collip, who fine-tuned the extraction process.

This raises many questions. Was the discovery of insulin inevitable? Was Banting a genius or simply someone who happened to be in the right place at the right time? Why was the prior contribution of the Romanian physiologist Nicholai Paulescu ignored? How important was the contribution of Macleod and Best?

Two editorials in the *Lancet* in 1923 questioned why the discovery of insulin had taken so long. The seductively simple critique went as follows: in 1869 Langerhans described his eponymous islets, in 1889 Minkowski and von Mehring produced diabetes in dogs by pancreatectomy, in 1891 Murray inaugurated the era of endocrine therapy with thyroid extract, and in 1893 Laguesse suggested that the islets of Langerhans produced something that controlled carbohydrate metabolism. How then could it have taken nearly thirty years to discover insulin?

The discovery of insulin: Banting, Macleod, Best, and Collip

After war service in Europe, Frederick Grant Banting (1891–1941) failed to get a surgical job at the prestigious Toronto Hospital for Sick Children and so set up as a doctor in London, Ontario. This was not a success, and to make ends meet he got a part-time job at the University of Toronto. In October 1920 he had to lecture the students on carbohydrate metabolism, about which he knew little. While preparing, he read an article about a man in whom a stone had blocked the pancreatic duct leading to atrophy of the digestive-enzyme-producing part of the gland but leaving the islets intact. This was hardly new, since it had been known for thirty years that this was what happened when the duct was tied in animals, but in his notebook Banting wrote:

Diabetus [sic]

Ligate pancreatic ducts of dog. Keeping dogs alive until acini degenerate leaving Islets.

Try to isolate the internal secretion of these to relieve glycosurea [sic][1]

Against the background of the fruitless attempts described in the previous chapter, it is not surprising that Macleod did not take Banting seriously. Macleod wrote: 'I found that Dr Banting had only a superficial textbook knowledge of the work that had been done and no familiarity with the methods by which such a problem could be investigated in the laboratory.'[2] Quite apart from Banting's ignorance, Macleod had lost interest in diabetes and was researching acid–base balance. Banting later said that during the first interview Macleod was so disinterested that he started reading letters on his desk. Nevertheless, he offered Banting a disused lab and two students, Charles Best (1899–1978) and Clark Noble (1900–78), who were to do alternate months. They tossed a coin to decide who should do the first month. Best 'won', but was so involved at the end of the month that Noble agreed that he should continue.

Banting needed an assistant, because he did not know how to measure blood sugar, and Macleod had wisely insisted on this as the end point of their experiments. During his research on the blood sugar of the turtle, Best had learned the new Lewis–Benedict method, which needed as little as 0.2 ml blood, whereas other methods needed 25 ml. Another stumbling block was that Banting had never done a pancreatectomy, an operation that at the time was used only in animal research. Macleod assisted at the first operation, but Banting and Best then worked alone, writing from time to time to Macleod, who replied with advice. In August 1921 they depancreatized two dogs and treated one with pancreatic extract leaving the other as a control. The untreated dog died in four days while the treated one remained well. Macleod was encouraged by their results but felt that the falls in blood sugar might be due to dilution or even normal fluctuations. He suggested further experiments, to which Banting objected violently and accused Macleod of trying to steal their thunder. Nevertheless, the experiments were done. When Macleod returned in October, he had a stormy interview with Banting, who threatened to go elsewhere if better facilities were not provided. At a departmental meeting on 14 November 1921 Banting and Best gave a preliminary presentation of their work. One important suggestion at this meeting was that the best way of showing that the extract worked would be if regular injections could prolong the life of diabetic dogs.

This was a logistic problem, because the duct-ligation method needed many dogs and a wait of seven weeks while the exocrine tissue degenerated. Banting's solution was to use foetal calf pancreas, which Best got from the local abattoir. The rationale, as Sobolev had suggested twenty years before, was that it contained a high proportion of islets in relation to exocrine tissue. An important breakthrough came in December, when Banting decided to use alcohol in making the extract (an idea Macleod had suggested some months before). It worked well and led them to wonder whether they could get a similar result with the more easily available adult beef pancreas. That they did must have been a surprise, because the original rationale for duct ligation was that the internal secretion

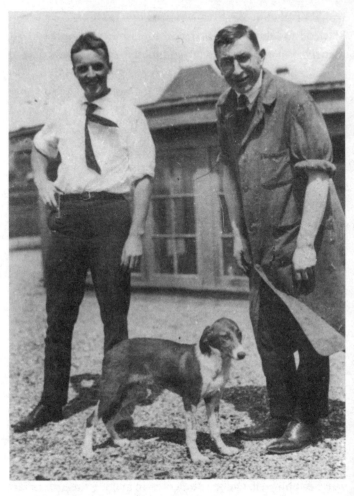

6. Charles Best (left) and Fred Banting (right) with one of the dogs used for a longevity experiment. (*Thomas Fisher Rare Book Library, Toronto*)

would be destroyed by pancreatic enzymes. In fact, although Macleod and others believed this, it had been known since 1875 that fresh pancreas did not break down proteins. The intact gland contains an inactive precursor trypsinogen, which is converted into the protein-dissolving enzyme trypsin only by contact with duodenal juice. Around this time Banting and Best were joined by a biochemist, Bert Collip (1892–1965)—more accurately, he was foisted on them by Macleod, who regarded him as a proper scientist. Collip had come on a Rockefeller fellowship and was studying the effect of pH on blood sugar. Later he was asked to help with the purification of insulin and made rapid progress, although afterwards he downplayed his role, suggesting that any biochemist could have done the same.

Some time in December 1921 Collip began making extracts from whole pancreas and, at Macleod's suggestion, tested them on rabbits. The extracts reduced the rabbit's blood sugar, and how far it fell was a useful and cheap way of telling how potent the extract was.

The first use of insulin (an extract made by Charles Best) on a human being was on 11 January 1922. The pancreatic extracts were relatively impure, and the house physician at Toronto General Hospital described what he injected into the buttocks of 14-year-old Leonard Thompson as '15 cc of thick brown muck'. Thompson had been on the Allen diet since 1919 and weighed only 65 lb (29.5 kg). After the injection, his blood sugar fell from 440 to 320 mg/dl (24.4 to 18.3 mmol/l), but no clinical benefit was seen. The experiment resumed on 23 January, when he was given Collip's extract, and now his blood sugar fell during one day from 520 mg/dl (29 mmol/l) to 120 mg/dl (6.7 mmol/l). He continued treatment for ten days with marked clinical improvement and complete elimination of glucose and ketones from his urine. Subsequently he lived a relatively normal life, although reliant on insulin injections, before dying of pneumonia in 1935.

The first clinical results were published in the March 1922 *Canadian Medical Association Journal*, where the authors reported that they had treated seven cases, Leonard Thompson being the only one described in detail. Dramatically the paper concluded:

(i) Blood sugar can be markedly reduced, even to normal values.

(ii) Glycosuria can be abolished.

(iii) The acetone bodies can be made to disappear from the urine.

(iv) The respiratory quotient shows evidence of increased utilization of carbohydrates.

(v) A definite improvement is observed in the general condition of these patients and, in addition, the patients themselves report a subjective sense of well being and increased vigor for a period following the administration of these preparations.[3]

The aftermath of this epoch-making discovery was scarred by bitter wrangling between the proponents, and disputes about the priority of the Romanian physiologist Paulescu. In the first six months of 1922 Banting could hardly bring himself to speak to Macleod, whom he later described as the most selfish man he had ever known. Banting turned the work of purifying insulin into a competition with Collip and, when he lost, was so ungracious that Collip at first refused to divulge the secret. He was also furious that Macleod, not Best, shared the Nobel prize with him.

Banting's position was invidious. He was revered as a maverick genius who had made the discovery of the century. Many Canadians thought he would be able to solve all medical mysteries if given the money. Although an orthopaedic surgeon, he was now regarded worldwide as an expert on diabetes. He did start a small diabetic clinic in Toronto but soon wound it up. He had decided that his future was going to be in research in anything but diabetes; he hoped to make another discovery as momentous as insulin but never did, despite having a large department. In 1938 he exasperatedly described his daily life:

> When I go in I find that it is not a lab but an office. There are a pile of letters to answer, phone numbers to call up, people waiting to have an interview, routine work that must be done. Some person wants me to give him some money, someone wants a signature, someone wants to know what to do about a friend of a great aunt's cousin who has a cancer, or who has gone insane. Someone has a cure for diarrhoea, cancer or anterior polyio myelitis [*sic*]. Some antivivisectionist damns. Some of the staff are sick or want a raise in salary or want a holiday. Some newspaperman wants an exclusive story, 'inside dope'. Someone has written an article and they wish it commented upon. Some member of the staff has an idea and they wish to discuss it. Some visitor from China, the USA, England has arrived and 'cannot visit Canada without seeing the distinguished discoverer of Insulin!'[4]

Best was also in a difficult position. He was only a medical student, but people thought of him as Banting's co-worker and peer. Unlike Banting, he was not immediately saddled with the title 'diabetes expert' and, after graduation, spent several years in England doing a PhD with the physiologist Henry Dale. Banting, who died in a plane crash in 1941, never credited Best with any ideas, and, in the words of Bliss, sometimes thought of him as 'his equal partner, at other times as a kind of officer's batman'.[5] By the last years of his life Banting disliked Best intensely and, just before he set off on his fatal flight said: 'If they ever give that chair of mine to that son of a bitch, Best, I'll roll over in my grave'. Best did get the chair and now became the chief spokesman for the view that he and Banting had discovered insulin on their own and been deprived of their full share of the glory by the machinations of Macleod, Collip, and their friends. As Michael Bliss has shown, Best literally rewrote the history of the discovery of insulin to put himself centre stage.

After returning to Edmonton, Collip qualified in medicine and in 1926 discovered parathyroid hormone. He made it up with Banting, and it was Collip who saw him off on his fatal flight. The person who has had the worst hearing at the bar of history is Macleod. On film he was portrayed by the actor Sir Ralph Richardson as dour and unattractive. He left Toronto in 1928 to become Regius Professor in Aberdeen and died in 1935.

One controversy that will never be resolved is whether the Romanian Nicholai Paulescu (1869–1931) should have shared the Nobel Prize. In contrast to the amateurs Banting and Best, Paulescu was a physiologist of international renown. His interest in diabetes began when he worked in Paris with Lancereaux. He went back to Bucharest in 1900 and became famous for his work on the pituitary gland. Having tried unsuccessfully to isolate the internal secretion of the pancreas in 1899, he did not try again until 1916. In his *Textbook of Medical Physiology*, published in French in Bucharest in 1919, he described a pancreatic extract that cured symptoms of diabetes in depancreatized dogs. He did more experiments in 1920, which were published in French journals in July and August 1921. These papers report a beautifully conceived and executed series of experiments, and in April 1922 he obtained a patent for 'Pancréine' but did not have the money or facilities to make it in large quantities.

When Paulescu heard about the award of the prize to the Canadians, he wrote to the President of the Nobel foundation citing his papers, which proved, in his words, 'that the treatment of diabetes was already discovered and nothing remained but its application in man'. In response he was sent a brochure, 'The Nobel Prizes of 1923'.

It is very unusual for Nobel Prizes to be awarded within two years of a discovery and to people nominated for the first time. What must have swayed the committee is that, when they made their decision, there was clear evidence that insulin was life-saving. Paulescu's scientific work was more impressive, but it was the Canadian group, with the commercial know-how of Eli Lilly, who had produced insulin in quantity.

Initial clinical experiences

Given the thirty-year history of false dawns since 1889, it is not surprising that the reports from Toronto were greeted with scepticism, especially in Europe. However, when Macleod presented the clinical results at the Association of American Physicians in May 1922, nobody seems to have doubted them, and he received a standing ovation. Insulin was supplied to American physicians in August 1922, and their experiences were published in ten papers in a special edition of Allen's *Journal of Metabolic Research* in 1923.

A picture is worth a thousand words, and the most impressive papers were those illustrated by 'before and after' photographs of children who had been resurrected by insulin. Best

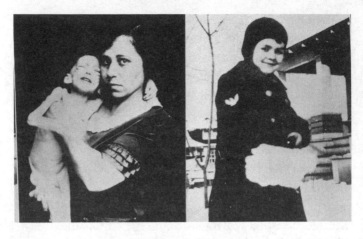

7. Ralph Major's patient Billy Leroy: before and after 79 days on insulin. (*Clendening Library, University of Kansas*)

known is that of Ralph Major's patient Billy Leroy. This 3-year-old boy had had diabetes for two years and weighed only 6.8 kilograms (15 lb). After three months on insulin his weight had doubled, and he was a normally active little boy.

Joslin's first patient to be treated with insulin was the 42-year-old Miss Mudge, who had had diabetes for five years, during which her weight had fallen from 72 to 33 kilograms. Her urine could not be kept sugar-free on any diet, and she was so weak that she had been out of her house only once in nine months before starting insulin in August 1922. Since then her weight had increased by 9 kilograms and, on 10 units of insulin and a diet of 25 grams of carbohydrate, she had a normal blood sugar before and after breakfast.

News of the discovery spread rapidly. According to *The Times* newspaper in August 1922, leading physicians in Canada and the USA agreed that the treatment had prolonged the lives of many sufferers and 'been effectual as a preventive in many cases'.[6] Outside North America the reaction of doctors ranged, according to the Spanish physician Rosend Carrasco-Formiguera (1892–1990), 'from extreme unwarranted optimism to more or less marked and equally unwarranted pessimism. There were those who expected a complete and definitive cure for diabetes. On the other hand there were those who claimed that insulin would only be effective—if at all—in special circumstances or in a small proportion of diabetic patients.'[7] However sceptical some doctors were, the press hailed insulin as a miracle. In April 1923 the local Nottingham paper, under the heading 'Certain diabetes cure: success of insulin a great medical triumph: all difficulties overcome', reported that:

> Complete success is at last attending the insulin treatment of diabetic patients and the discovery is regarded in medical circles as one of the great scientific achievements of the age...A remarkable cure has just been effected at the St Thomas's Hospital in the case of a man who had contracted the disease, hitherto considered fatal, as a result of shock after being torpedoed. His body wasted away almost to a skeleton and his life was despaired of. But soon after Christmas he was admitted to the hospital, treated with insulin, and now he cycles up to London every day from his home in Surrey.[8]

Then, as now, readers must have found it difficult to distinguish truth from fiction. A week earlier, under the heading 'Simple consumption cure: Australian doctor's successful treatment', the same newspaper had reported a cure for TB that consisted of blowing tubercle bacilli up the nose. It also carried an item about injections to revive the dead. Personal testimony was more reliable, and in August 1923 a layman wrote to *The Times* with his experience of the new treatment:

I was a bit of a sceptic about insulin. One hears of a number of sensational recoveries...I had tried two pancreatic preparations and both had failed. Thus it was in no optimistic vein that I submitted to the course of punctures and injections and blood tests. The prospect rather bored me, but I had the chance...On the second day the miracle was accomplished. The tests declared that the poison was out of my system. For weeks and months, the most vigorous diet had failed to evict it...the ding-dong battle (the inevitable return of sugar and acetone when insulin is omitted for a day) is the meaning of insulin for me at the moment, and the fact that six weeks ago it saved my life. The enemy was well within the defences. Insulin is a force of magical activity, but its effects are not permanent.[9]

Commercial production

In North America the University of Toronto gave the pharmaceutical company Eli Lilly exclusive rights to produce and sell insulin for a year. Lilly was to give it free to selected clinicians, have all batches tested in Toronto, and assign the patent for improvements to the University. In October 1922 the Danish Nobel Prize winner August Krogh (1874–1949) was lecturing in the USA and asked Macleod if he could test insulin in his country—his wife Marie had developed diabetes a year earlier, so he had a personal as well as a professional interest. Production in Denmark began in December 1922, and within a year Danish insulin was being exported to several European countries. In July 1922 the University of Toronto asked the British Medical Research Council (MRC) to accept the patent rights. The Council, set up in 1911 for research into tuberculosis, was reluctant, but the clamour from physicians and the public meant that they had to do something, and their involvement offered the opportunity to 'exercise a moral control of manufacturers and induce them to submit to a system of supervision, as regards this product, which the law does not enable the Council at present to enforce'.[10] The reason for the MRC's concern was that, in England until 1925, any drug could be advertised and marketed as a cure for any disease, even if it was completely ineffective.

One unforeseen consequence was that 'enquiring, appealing, often heartrending letters arrived by the sack' at the MRC offices. Approaches were made to drug companies, and the first British insulin was supplied to hospitals in April 1923.

Getting to grips with the new treatment

Insulin was totally different from existing medicines, its use raised as many questions as it answered, and every part of every answer raised more questions.

Newspapers led the public to believe that insulin was a cure and doctors did think it might rest the insulin-producing cells and allow them to regenerate. This was not irrational; the kidneys could recover after acute glomerulonephritis and the lungs after lobar pneumonia, so why not the pancreas? It therefore made sense to try to nurse the islets back to health by rest. Initial experience was encouraging; patients often needed large doses of insulin at first, but a month or two later these could be halved or quartered (what was later called the honeymoon effect—that is, something transient). By 1925 it was clear that regeneration did not occur and that insulin was a life sentence.

Attempts were made to give insulin by mouth, inhalation, rectally, and through the skin, but it soon became obvious that it had to be injected. Hypodermic injections had been used by doctors since the 1850s and were the method of choice for morphine addicts (often, according to the *Lancet*, 'members of the weaker sex of the upper or middle class'[11]). Nevertheless, the idea that ordinary people should be allowed to, or would be able to, inject themselves seemed to many doctors outrageous, perhaps because it would transfer power to the patient, which to some extent it did. In the event, injections were not the stumbling block predicted by many doctors. Robin (R. D.) Lawrence (1892–1968) of King's College Hospital, London, himself a diabetic saved by insulin, made his patients give their own injections and claimed that few, if any, had difficulties after the first week.

Whether general practitioners should use insulin was debated at the British Medical Association in 1923, where Banting said that, when patients in Toronto left hospital, they were thoroughly au fait with the insulin routine, and a detailed letter was sent to the GP. Several North American hospitals began courses for family doctors in 1923. The response of English physicians was ambivalent, in that in their writings they encouraged GPs to use insulin but stressed how powerful and dangerous it was. Given the low level of sophistication in general practice in England, the average GP probably agreed with a Dr Sanderson, who wrote to the *BMJ*: 'Whatever may be the benefits conferred on the diabetic by insulin, there seemed little doubt that it bade fair to bring many practitioners to a premature grave so multitudinous, bewildering and worrying were the problems involved.'[12]

He was not alone. In Australia similar concerns were voiced by the editor of the *Medical Journal of Australia*, who attacked insulin as a dangerous and unproven remedy and suggested hyperbolically that it was too potent to be used outside hospitals and that 'no doubt hundreds of diabetics will be hastened to their graves'.[13]

For patients the index of success of insulin was obvious; freedom from thirst and excessive urination and gain of weight and energy. However, many physicians believed in the more demanding target of normal blood-sugar levels. Chapters in two popular English medical textbooks recommended that the urine should always be sugar free and the fasting blood sugar between 80 and 120 mg/dl (4.4–6.7 mmol/l). Most American physicians agreed, the most uncompromising being Joslin, who wrote in 1928: 'Glycosuria is not only tolerated but encouraged by several physicians highly skilled in the treatment of diabetes. Even 20 grams of glucose are allowed in the urine by design. To this plan of treatment I am emphatically opposed…success in the treatment of diabetic children lies in keeping their urine sugar-free. If sugar appears, a penalty follows.'[14]

Most people with diabetes feel well, irrespective of whether their blood sugar is 5, 10, or 15 mmol/l. Furthermore, most found it impossible to keep their blood sugar constantly normal and would have agreed with Lawrence, who suggested that trying to do so made their life unnecessarily hard without obvious benefit. The downside of a sugar free urine at all times was that it increased the probability of the novel condition of hypoglycaemia or abnormally low blood sugar. Before insulin, physiologists had produced hypoglycaemia by removing the liver in experimental animals, but it had been reported in humans (with Addison's disease) fewer than half a dozen times. It was first recognized in Toronto when a lab man told Clark Noble that rabbits used to standardize the strength of insulin died overnight with convulsions. Noble found that their blood sugar was very low and credited Macleod with the idea of injecting them with glucose, which led to instant recovery. This 'resurrection' of unconscious rabbits became a *pièce de resistance* for visitors to the lab.

The experience of treating hypoglycaemia in human beings was equally dramatic. Carrasco-Formiguera remembered it in a 4-year-old boy he treated in 1923:

> The [insulin] treatment was carried out in a small hospital where the boy was under the continuous surveillance of his mother. One day she suddenly burst into my office telling me that her son was dying. I rushed to see the boy and was myself reassured when I saw that, although he was in a coma, he showed the typical hypoglycaemic syndrome, which I had never seen in human beings, but about which I had read very much. I slowly administered an i.v. glucose injection. Even though, from my readings and from my experience with rabbits, I was prepared for what followed, I was as amazed as the mother when the boy opened his eyes and said something sensible, even before the injection had been completed. And I was certainly as elated as the mother when less than half an hour later the boy was happily playing.[15]

In the 1923, the Toronto physicians Andrew Almon Fletcher and Walter Campbell gave a vivid description of the varied effects of low blood sugar in humans:

> The initial symptom may be a feeling of nervousness or tremulousness, sometimes a feeling of excessive hunger, at other times a feeling of weakness or a sense of goneness. The level at which a patient becomes aware of the fall in blood sugar is fairly constant for that individual, although this is not always the case...[as the blood sugar falls further]...the feeling of nervousness may become definite anxiety, excitement or even emotional upset. The feeling of tremulousness is possibly a form of incoordination. Patients have shown a loss of power to perform fine movements with their fingers...Much

more severe manifestations are observed with further lowering of the blood sugar. Marked excitement, emotional
instability, sensory and motor aphasia, dysarthria, delirium,
disorientation, confusion have all been seen.[16]

Soon hypoglycaemia was being compared to drunkenness.
Otto Leyton told of one of his patients who, during a meal,
pressed his friends to help themselves to more pepper. Then
in a loud voice, he insulted his wife, who, realising that he was
hypoglycaemic, asked him to take some sugar. He replied that,
of course she wanted him to take sugar, something the doctor
had specifically forbidden, so that she could get rid of him and
marry someone else. Eventually he was forced to take sugar,
became normal within a few minutes, and had no recollection
of what had happened.

Coma that was due to low blood sugar (hypoglycaemic
coma) was a new disease, and what doctors understood by the
term 'diabetic coma' was ketoacidosis. Some of the most dramatic effects of insulin were seen in these patients. In 1923 Nellis
Foster (1875–1933) of Philadelphia treated fifteen coma patients
with insulin, of whom eight recovered, the first survivors he had
ever seen. All but two of Joslin's first thirty-three coma cases
treated with insulin between 1923 and 1925 survived.

The size of the first dose of insulin for coma in Joslin's unit was
based on the doctors' estimate of how long the patient would
have lived without it—having seen so many deaths, this was
presumably one of their clinical skills. Thus, 'if the expectation
of life is twenty-four hours, one would inject 20 units and repeat
every hour until clinical improvement is evident; if the expectation is twelve hours one would inject 40 units and repeat the
dose in the same manner'.[17] One of the most striking features of
ketoacidosis is the dehydration shown by the parched tongue,

inelastic skin, and sunken eyeballs. Nowadays one or two litres of salt solution would be given intravenously during the first hour, but in the 1920s it was thought that intravenous fluids would strain the heart, and fluids were given either subcutaneously or rectally. Stimulation of the heart was regarded as essential with subcutaneous caffeine injections for the first few hours, often supplemented by a coffee enema.

It has often been suggested that insulin immediately revolutionized the outlook for pregnant diabetic women. In fact, what it did was to reduce maternal mortality from 50 per cent to around 3 per cent. The outlook for the baby remained poor, with two series in 1933 reporting foetal mortalities of 64 per cent and 41 per cent. The results were so discouraging that women on insulin were advised not to get pregnant, and sterilization was actively encouraged.

Insulin in the non-diabetic

Brown-Séquard's testicular extract and thyroid extract were tried in almost every disease in the 1890s, and insulin went through a similar trajectory in the 1920s. One of its most striking effects was weight gain, and it was used to stimulate appetite in tuberculosis and 'in the insane refusing food'. Good results were reported when it was applied locally to wounds, and one of the first of many papers in the next forty years reporting its use in healing bedsores was published in 1930.

Its most notorious use was the insulin coma therapy, which was claimed to lead to a remission in 70 per cent of schizophrenics. This became so popular that by the late 1930s most English psychiatric hospitals had a dedicated insulin unit. Large doses of insulin were given, leading to what one observer called 'a frenzy of disorganized activity' of the whole nervous system, although eventually the patient woke from his coma with 'no trace of the neurologic storm through which he had passed.' Having an active treatment appealed to psychiatrists, whose previous function had been primarily to act as custodians to schizophrenics, who formed two-thirds of the permanent mental-hospital population. How effective it was is uncertain, and complication rates were high. A particular problem was irreversible coma due to hypoglycaemic brain damage, also occasionally seen in diabetic patients. After the introduction of the first anti-psychotic drug, chlorpromazine, in 1952, insulin coma was phased out.

How did the new insulin-dependent diabetics manage?

How insulin affected the everyday lives of those now depend-ent on daily injections is hard to discover, because the scientific literature concentrated on the practical aspects of therapy, and the few accounts by patients stressed their miraculous resurrec-tion and gratitude to Banting.

Most newly diagnosed diabetics in England, America, and Germany were admitted to hospitals or nursing homes for a week or more to start insulin. A few started treatment as an outpatient, usually because they could not afford anything else. For example, in 1925 an American physician described a man who had been started on insulin and 'given a working knowl-edge of how to take care of himself within three hours'. Similar cases were reported from Germany. In 1929 a Boston doctor described forty-eight patients 'of average intelligence' who had started insulin as outpatients, of whom 80 per cent managed well. Nevertheless, starting treatment as an outpatient remained very much the exception for the next fifty years.

The equipment that patients were advised to have was two syringes (one a spare), six 25-gauge hypodermic needles ⅜ inch long, a cylindrical glass tube, and a wood block to stand it in. The syringe (with needle on) was placed in the tube, which was filled with alcohol, and corked to prevent evaporation. Later, metal or Bakelite cases for storing the syringe in alcohol were produced. Syringes were glass and were supposed to be boiled before each injection. Needles had to be resharpened regularly with a stone. Other innovations followed as the demand for syringes grew. The Yale Luer-Lok, introduced in 1925, stopped the needle coming off or damaging the end of the syringe. Apart from breakage from boiling, other syringe problems were jamming of the plunger by residues from the methylated spirits in which it was kept and loosening of the plunger, leading to inaccuracies in dosing.

In England the first strength of insulin marketed was 20 units/ml (later called single strength), and syringes were made with 20 marks per millilitre, so that one mark equalled one unit. When 40- and 80-units/ml (double and quadruple strength) insulins were introduced in the 1930s, the old syringe was retained, so that marks on the syringe and units no longer corresponded. This caused confusion, because, depending on which strength of insulin was being used, a mark could be 1, 2, or 4 units, and some patients quoted their dose as 10 units when they meant 10 marks of 80 u/cc insulin—that is, 40 units. In the USA, and less commonly in Europe, syringes were made with dual scales for 40- and 80-strength insulin, which caused halving or doubling of the dose if the patient inadvertently used the wrong scale. These problems were not solved until a single strength of 100

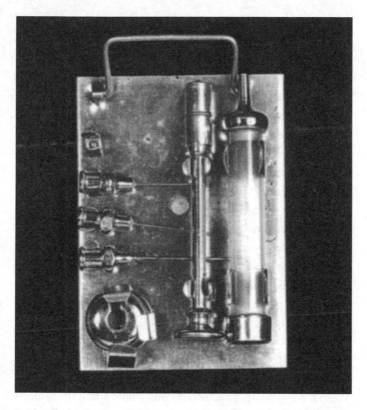

8. Hypodermic syringe of the type used for insulin in the 1920s. (*Wellcome Library, London*)

units/ml was introduced in the 1980s, with a standard syringe in which units and marks again corresponded.

In the 1920s there was only one type of insulin (a clear solution called soluble in England and regular in America), and most patients injected twice daily. Because preparations were relatively impure, allergic reactions (mainly itchy lumps) at injection sites were common. By contrast, infections were, and have continued to be, rare—in 1922–3 Joslin recorded none in over 5,000 injections, and I saw only two in thirty years of clinical practice.

Diet (usually low carbohydrate and high fat) was rigidly prescribed, and patients were taught to weigh their food, although most abandoned their scales after a few years, claiming to be able to gauge the amount by eye. Progress was charted with Benedict's test, in which urine was boiled with a copper solution; if there was no sugar, the mixture remained blue, and, if there was a lot, it turned brick red. Blood sugar was only measured, if at all, at clinic visits.

Even before insulin, patient education was regarded by some physicians as an integral part of treatment, and classes were organized by hospitals in America and Germany, but not, as far as I can discover, in most English hospitals, where education was usually given by the ward sister. Patient handbooks had been available before insulin, but the market expanded greatly after 1923, with the best known in England being Lawrence's *The Diabetic Life: Its Control by Diet and Insulin*. Many proved enduring best-sellers. Lawrence's reached its fifteenth edition in 1944 and Joslin's its eighth in 1959.

How people on insulin were advised to order their new lives depended on their physician. Some advised a quiet life, while other expected them to go back to their previous jobs. When a Scottish doctor reviewed one year's experience of insulin in 1925, he reported:

> One man continues to work as a bricklayer and loses no more time than his fellows. Another works all night in a printing office. Two carry on successfully as commercial travellers. One is at work as a tramway conductor. Two boys attend school regularly. The majority of the women are at home,

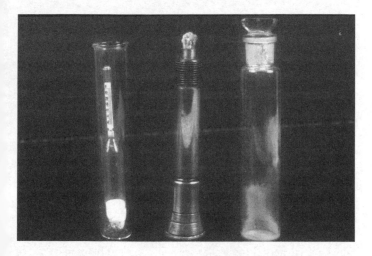

9. Urine testing kit from the 1930s. From left to right are test tube and hydrometer to measure the specific gravity of the urine, brass spirit lamp (centre) and container for Benedict's solution.

and are quite fit for their housework...two are in nursing, both in rather strenuous employment.[18]

The first professional sportsman to write an account of how diabetes affected his career was the American tennis player Billy Talbert (1918–99). He developed diabetes in 1928 and describes how, during his childhood, he lived in dread of a positive Benedict's test either at home or at his clinic visits—adults, in his view, would have interpreted this as evidence of cheating. When he entered his first tournament at the age of 16 he explained:

> I had to go on and explain [to the wife of the organizer] about the diabetes. It took some talking on my part to persuade her that I was physically fit to play in her husband's tournament and even then she kept eyeing me as if she expected me to

drop at any moment. Her husband relieved her—and dis-
comfited me—by promising to have a doctor at the courts.[19]

His later tennis career was very successful. He is remembered
winning the US doubles title four times, including a final in 1946
that lasted for seventy-four games. Before the Second World War
many employers would not knowingly have employed someone
with diabetes. Those on insulin were perceived as a liability, since
they might go into a hypoglycaemic coma at any time. Also diabetics were thought to be at risk of devastating infections from
a simple scratch and might have to have an amputation from
what, for the non-diabetic, would have been a trivial accident. In
1938 Lawrence wrote that 'a person with diabetes cannot enter
any Governmental or similar service, is barred from all types of
employment which are pensionable, and is liable to find himself
discharged when his private employer knows of his diabetes'.[20] In
fact, when surveys of diabetic workers were done in the 1950s, it
turned out that their absenteeism rate was no different from that
of 'healthy' workers. Whether those on insulin should be allowed
to drive cars, lorries, or buses was discussed from time to time. In
a radio broadcast in England in 1948, the doctor narrator said:

> The legal position is that diabetics can hold driving licences
> and do not have to reveal in applying for them that they are
> diabetics. This puts a great responsibility on them to see that
> they are not a danger on the road. A few unstable diabetics
> who are particularly liable to reactions should not drive at all
> and it's their doctor's business to tell them so.[21]

However, whatever the doctor advised, the person with diabetes
could continue to drive and in the 1950s and 1960s could have
quoted surveys showing that diabetic drivers actually had fewer
accidents than other drivers.

Well into the second half of the twentieth century clinicians in most countries expected patients to be passive and did not encourage them to participate in their own treatment or even to ask questions; there is no reason why this should have been any different for those with diabetes, and it was not. Not only were they high and mighty, but the London teaching-hospital physicians who became the experts in insulin treatment in 1923 had very strong backgrounds in biochemistry and appeared to be clinicians almost by default. Their obituaries are revealing: George Graham (St Bartholomew's) 'may not have been the world's greatest clinician'; Hugh Maclean (St Thomas's) was a chemical pathologist until appointed to the newly established chair of medicine in 1921 'in spite of his relatively limited clinical experience'; Otto Leyton (The London) was a reserved and dilettante figure who finished his ward round in half an hour and then 'treated his clerks to an interesting but entirely theoretical discourse'.[22]

In the 1920s diabetic clinics were set up in Edinburgh, at King's College Hospital, London, and in a few other places, but most patients were followed up in ordinary general medical clinics. As the number of diabetics increased, physicians found it too time-consuming to look after them, and many diabetic clinics were set up to get rid of these unwanted cases rather than to give them expert care. Since GPs had in effect been frozen out of diabetes care, hospital clinics soon became very overcrowded. In 1945 a Sheffield doctor described one clinic:

> It has been the practice to let the patients attend periodically. They arrive in the fasting state in a large outpatient hall, and sit on benches which are usually overcrowded on clinic mornings (60 to 70 patients may attend). They queue slowly to have their weights recorded and then have venous blood drawn for blood sugar estimations.[23]

Thirty years later this would have been an accurate description of the clinic that I inherited as a new consultant in Nottingham. The one at the other Nottingham hospital was, according to one of my colleagues, 'run in more military fashion by a consultant noted for his custom of writing "W.O.T." in red ink on the notes of unsatisfactory patients. "W.O.T." stood for "Waste of Time", and so indeed it was.' [24]

A lack of empathy and common ground between doctors and patients partly explains the unsatisfactory outcomes described in the next chapter.

IV

—∞∞∞—

THE DARK AGES

In the decade after the discovery of insulin, doctors were optimistic about the future—at least for young patients. In 1930 Frederick Allen proclaimed that diabetes had been mastered and that every patient could be expected to live out his full natural lifetime. For Allen and his friend Joslin, this would be achieved if blood sugars were controlled by hard work, perseverance, and intelligence. Such views were by no means held by all doctors and formed the basis for the long-running control and complications debate. Two developments in the 1930s—long-acting insulins and free diets—polarized the controversy.

Long-acting insulins

The need for a longer-acting preparation became obvious in the late 1920s, when purification of ordinary or soluble insulin shortened its action and meant that many people needed an injection before each meal and, most inconveniently, one at 3 a.m. Attempts had been made in the 1920s to prolong the action of insulin, but all failed, and the first practical long-acting insulin was protamine insulinate, made in 1936 by Hans Christian Hagedorn (1888–1971) at Nordisk Insulinlaboratorium in Copenhagen. His aim was to produce a solid compound of insulin that dissolved gradually after injection. Many additives were tried before his co-worker Norman Jensen suggested substances called protamines found in the nucleus of sperm. The one finally chosen was from the rainbow trout. Studies on patients in his hospital showed that protamine insulin got rid of the sharp peak of blood sugar seen when ordinary insulin ran out three or four hours after injection; it lasted twice as long and was particularly useful to control blood sugars overnight. Hagedorn gave supplies to Joslin in America and Lawrence in England; both wrote eulogistic articles but agreed that ordinary insulin was also necessary to control the blood-sugar rise after meals.

More long-acting preparations were introduced in the next fifteen years. Protamine zinc insulin (PZI) was developed in Toronto in 1936 and lasted more than twenty-four hours. To many doctors its selling point was that treatment with one injection a day was now possible, and Lawrence described it as the 'practitioner's insulin for choice'. For what were at the time called mild cases (that is, type 2 diabetics) PZI alone was often enough, but, for more severe cases, soluble insulin had to be added to prevent glucose peaks after breakfast. Patients and doctors soon discovered that, on the new insulins, hypoglycaemic symptoms were slower in onset and less obvious to the patient. The Mayo clinic physician Russell Wilder (1885–1959) had personal experience. In May 1936 he went from Minnesota to a meeting in Kansas City with his assistant Dr Randall Sprague and dietitian Miss Nelson, both of whom had diabetes. On the second evening Dr Sprague could not be found and was eventually located wandering in the streets distractedly 'in a delayed reaction from protamine insulin'. On the drive home they stopped at a hotel, where Miss Nelson was unable to write her name in the register because of hypoglycaemia. It took some persuasion to convince the proprietor that she was not drunk! Wilder later quoted one of his patients on PZI as saying, 'I don't have diabetes any more, I have insulin reactions.'[1] Many patients rejected long-acting insulins. One was the chest physician Charles Fletcher (1911–95), who developed diabetes in 1940, an eventful year in which he also got married and gave the world's first penicillin injection. He found PZI

> socially intolerable. It demands an evening meal at a fixed time which is often impracticable, especially after going to a theatre or in foreign countries where dinner may be very late…At my wife's suggestion I started doing what the normal pancreas does and went over to three injections of soluble insulin daily before my main meals, supplementing the evening dose with a little isophane to cover the next early morning. I take extra insulin supplements to control unusual hyperglycaemia.[2]

One injection of insulin a day was attractive but one a month would have been even better. In 1948 a Chilean doctor made pellets of PZI and cholesterol which were implanted in 7 patients. Amazingly, a 10-year old child received 16,850 units in a single implantation. The suggestion was that about 1 per cent was absorbed per day so that an implant would last 80–100 days. The doctor concluded optimistically that 'this new way of administering insulin will not only abolish daily injections but also may achieve better results'.[3] Nothing more was heard of it.

Other long-acting insulins were globin, in which the retarding agent came from ox blood, and surfen, in which the retarding agent was a substance used as an antiseptic. Globin was little used, but surfen insulins survived in Germany until the 1980s. What became the most popular insulin worldwide was NPH (Neutral Protamine Hagedorn or isophane), which was developed at Nordisk in Copenhagen in 1940. The Lente series, a combination of insulin and zinc, were made by Novo laboratories in 1952. How long Lente insulins lasted depended on the physical state of the particles, amorphous ones being shorter acting than crystals. There were three preparations; The fastest, Semilente was only amorphous particles, the longest, Ultralente, was purely crystalline and the most popular, Lente, was a 30:70 mixture of Semilente and Ultralente. It was claimed that 85 to 90 per cent of patients could be controlled—that is, kept symptom free—on a single daily injection of Lente, and glowing reports, standard for any new insulin then as in the twenty-first century, followed in English and American medical journals. Most patients and doctors were impressed by the convenience of an insulin that could be given once a day and then forgotten. Unfortunately this, combined with the free-diet movement, led to three decades in which poor glucose control was the rule rather than the exception.

An epidemic of complications

In the pre-insulin era retinopathy occurred only in older diabetics and was thought to be due to artherosclerosis. Particularly influential for this theory was a survey in 1921 at the Mayo Clinic, where Wilder and the ophthalmologist Henry Wagener found retinal lesions in middle-aged or elderly diabetics but not in any of eighty young patients (who, since they had a fatal disease, had all had diabetes for less than five years). They concluded that retinal damage did not occur in 'severe' diabetes but only in the 'mild and chronic' form, where it was accompanied by hardening of the arteries. This paradigm changed in 1934, when they found young patients (some of whom had now had diabetes for ten years or more) with retinal haemorrhages but no other clinical evidence of vascular disease. They concluded that diabetes alone injured the small blood vessels of the retina. How this damage was caused they did not know, and what was confusing was that it was seen in cases of mild diabetes (those managed by diet alone) as frequently as in severe diabetes (those on insulin). Nobody yet realized that insulin had converted the acute fatal form of diabetes into something more like the chronic form.

Further evidence that diabetes alone could cause organ damage was the 1936 discovery by Paul Kimmelsteil (1900–70) and Clifford Wilson (1906–97) of a new type of kidney disease. Their eight middle-aged diabetic patients lost a large amount of protein in their urine and had gross oedema, a clinical picture known as the nephrotic syndrome. What was new was the microscopic appearance of the kidney, where there were large nodules in the glomeruli (intercapillary glomerulosclerosis). After the Second World War it became clear that this kidney disease could also affect the young, and there were increasingly frequent reports of diabetics who had been saved by insulin as children only to succumb to kidney failure in their 20s and 30s. Fifty of Joslin's child patients who had started insulin before 1929 were followed up in 1949, when a third had died at an average age of 25, after having had diabetes for an average of 17.6 years. One half had died of kidney failure and the other half of tuberculosis and other infections. Markers of early kidney disease were protein in the urine (albuminuria) and high blood pressure, and these harbingers of future trouble were found in most of the survivors. In the experience of the Joslin group, only 2 per cent of deaths of young diabetic patients before 1937 were due to kidney disease, but, of those who died between 1944 and 1950, more than half had advanced kidney disease. Results in Europe were equally bad. In 1955 all of eighty-seven Swiss children had signs of kidney disease after sixteen years of diabetes, and after twenty-one years all had died. Most young people with diabetic kidney disease also had severe retinopathy and many became blind—by the mid 1950s diabetes was the commonest cause of new blindness in people under the age of 50.

Kidney failure and blindness were presumably unanticipated by patients, and we know little about how they and their families reacted to them. This gap has been partly filled by Chris Feudtner in his book *Bittersweet*, which contains histories of Joslin's patients in the 1940s and 1950s. One was a boy who developed diabetes at the age of 4 and was found to have retinopathy, albuminuria, and hypertension on routine examination at the age of 27, when he felt well and was working full time. Since these 'invisible' complications were untreatable, he was not told about them, but a year later his mother wrote to Joslin: 'He is working but acts so weary, I would like to know what tonic he could take.' Joslin replied that strict control of the diabetes was the best tonic. A few months later, over the course of one week, he became blind in both eyes and wrote to his doctors asking: 'What am I supposed to do? What can I expect? If I can't work, how can I live? Please tell me what to do.' There was no answer, and in 1956 he died aged 33 from a heart attack shortly after a mid-thigh amputation for gangrene of his foot.[4]

Many young diabetics also developed the type of nerve damage that Pavy and others had described in the nineteenth century. The commonest manifestation was pain in the legs, but it could affect any part of the body, from the pupils to the feet. Patients were recorded as having intractable diarrhoea (diabetic diarrhoea), vomiting from paralysis of nerves to the stomach (gastroparesis), and disintegration of the ankle joint (Charcot joint), and many, if not most, men became sexually impotent.

Such devastating cases were being increasingly reported in the medical literature in the late 1940s and early 1950s, but they were not publicized in the lay press, presumably to avoid spreading despair and despondency and puncturing the myth that insulin had solved the problem of diabetes and allowed diabetic children, in Joslin's words, 'to live virtually indefinitely'. The British Diabetic Association (founded in 1935) produced a quarterly *Diabetic Journal* for its lay members, but no issue from 1940 to 1960 mentions complications, probably because of the dominance of paternalistic doctors in the organization. Most articles were triumphalist and patronizing, telling the stories of diabetics who held down busy and responsible jobs, had been on climbing holidays in the Alps, and so on. The main aim of the *Journal* seems to have been to dispel the idea that people with diabetes were in any way invalids.

The rising tide of complications fuelled a debate in medical journals about whether they could be prevented by controlling blood-sugar levels. Many physicians advocated this, on the basis that, if nature had ordained a blood sugar under 8 mmol/l as the normal state, it must be best. The argument became inextricably mixed up with the emotive subject of free diets.

Free diets

In 1923, when insulin was still very expensive, the diet was altered little from the extremely restricted one that had kept people alive long enough to benefit from its discovery. Essentially a small carbohydrate intake meant a low dose of insulin. At the end of the 1920s some physicians in the USA and Canada introduced high-carbohydrate diets, which, contrary to general expectations, led to a reduction in insulin dose. Other advantages cited were that high-carbohydrate diets were more palatable and cheaper. Also patients were more likely to stick to the diet, because they did not feel constantly hungry. Nevertheless, many doctors continued to prescribe a low-carbohydrate diet, because of an engrained belief that carbohydrate was bad for diabetics and concern that diabetic patients were untrustworthy and that, if given an inch, would take a mile.

The introduction of so-called free diets during the 1930s caused controversy and acrimony for nearly thirty years. The names associated with this movement were Karl Stolte (1881–1951) of Breslau, Adolf Lichtenstein (1884–1950) of Stockholm, and most notoriously Edward Tolstoi (1897–1983) of New York.

Stolte did advise his patients to eat a normal diet, but they were also expected to keep their urine sugar free. This was achieved by an injection before every meal, the dose depending on the size of the meal—a regimen that was not reintroduced in Germany or elsewhere until the 1980s. Stolte was opposed by Gerhardt Katsch (1887–1961), the unrivalled leader of diabetology in Germany. His style was extremely rigid, and he discouraged his patients from altering insulin doses. He also introduced hospital admissions of 4–6 weeks every year for 'stabilization', which became standard practice in Germany and to a lesser extent other European countries. Another of Stolte's opponents was Ferdinand Bertram (1894–1960), author of a best-selling patient handbook, who actively discouraged urine testing and advised a single daily injection of long-acting insulin.

Tolstoi, who worked in New York, started using protamine insulin as a once-daily injection in the late 1930s, but his patients found that trying to keep the urine sugar free led to warningless hypoglycaemia. Two abandoned their diet and reported that, in spite of continuously having sugar in their urine, they felt well. During two months in hospital they passed up to 100 grams of sugar in twenty-four hours, but, according to Tolstoi, had a normal urinary volume and no diabetic symptoms. He therefore decided to let all his patients eat what they liked and see what happened. He described the result:

> They are in good health, in a state of social and economic usefulness, and infections are no more frequent than in the average individual. All these patients enjoy their freedom as there appeared no necessity for careful dietary management, and it is not necessary for them to carry their insulin and syringe with them. They administer insulin to themselves in the morning and then put the equipment away until the following morning. These patients are not singled out as a group, apart from their fellow men, and their habits of living approximate the normal.[5]

To the criticism that they would develop complications, he pointed out that only 8 per cent of Joslin's juvenile onset patients avoided retinopathy and kidney disease in spite of sermons about the importance of 'chemical control'. To Tolstoi, quality of life was all-important, and, according to him, Joslin's patients 'do not enjoy life nor have the freedom of people who live like normal human beings'.

The conflict of opinion between Tolstoi and Joslin was also reflected among paediatricians. Robert Jackson (b. 1909) of Iowa and Adolf Lichtenstein of Stockholm were the polar opposites. Jackson was, from 1940, a fervent advocate of 'physiological' control in children, because, as he told me, 'it was the way nature intended it'. His child patients were treated with soluble insulin before each meal and globin at night. Urine was tested four times a day for glucose and ketones, and parents kept a detailed daily record of these tests, diet, and activities.

Lichtenstein believed that a rigid diet harmed mental development and social adjustment. Children attending his clinic ate the same food as their siblings and were allowed some sugar and sweets. Semantic problems had always bedevilled the free-diet debate, but Lichtenstein emphasized that what he was proposing was normal balanced fare, unlike the high-fat, low-carbohydrate diets prescribed by many diabetologists. Unlike Tolstoi, he was not prepared to accept totally uncontrolled hyperglycaemia. After his death, Lichtenstein's colleagues published a survey of his patients. There was, as everywhere else, an increasing incidence of complications with increasing duration of disease, but it was no higher than among patients treated with weighed and measured diets in other clinics. Free diets were also used for adults in Sweden and one of their strongest advocates was Bertil Söderling (1905–89), who occupied a special position as the radio doctor giving weekly broadcasts on medical matters— Charles Hill held this position in England at the same time. Söderling's daughter had diabetes, and, after she developed severe complications, he is said to have regretted deeply the line he had defended so strongly.

In the heat of battle it seems to have been assumed that the beliefs of physicians influenced the degree of control achieved by their patients. In 1953 Frederick Allen lamented:

The vast majority of cases in the United States and still more in other countries are not controlled in any real sense. The ignorance and carelessness of patients can often rightly be blamed; nevertheless, the majority are largely influenced by the attitude and personality of the physician. Inadequately trained physicians are apt to treat diabetes in the easiest way.[6]

Many physicians in the USA and Europe professed to believe in good control. When Samuel Beaser (1910–2006) questioned American diabetes specialists in 1951, half said they asked their patients to aim for normal fasting blood sugar, and hardly any disregarded blood sugars altogether. In 1953 in England a survey of eighty-one physicians in charge of diabetic clinics found that twenty-six aimed for normal blood sugars and thirty-eight for mild hyperglycaemia. When asked whether high blood sugars caused complications, thirty were sure they did, six thought definitely not, and the rest sat on the fence. Only half, irrespective of their beliefs about control, encouraged patients to test their urine at home. What probably sowed doubt in physicians' minds were the exceptional cases: a lab man at King's, whose control was thought by Lawrence to be excellent, went blind, while others with habitually poor control seemed to escape.

Many studies in the decade after the Second World War tried to discover whether blood-sugar control and complications were connected. Most had serious design flaws, but the main problem was the impossibility of assessing glucose control accurately when all there was to go on was the patient's record of urine tests and three or four clinic blood sugars a year.

Maintaining normal blood sugars, even if one's physician recommended it, was not easy. Until the introduction of Clinitest by the Ames Company in 1944, urine glucose was measured with

Benedict's solution and the paraphernalia of spirit lamps and spurting test tubes. The innovative feature of Clinitest was that the tablet contained caustic soda, which generated heat and did away with the need for a spirit lamp, thus making the test more convenient and portable. Whether the patient used Benedict's or Clinitest, the end result was the same—blue (no sugar) was 'good' and orange or red (sugar) was 'bad'. A serious disadvantage of urine tests was that they did not accurately reflect blood glucose at the time of sampling, because of the delay between the formation of urine and its passage and the variability of renal threshold for glucose from patient to patient. Such imperfections were glossed over, and patients were expected to bring a sheaf of records to their clinic visits. Whose benefit these were for is difficult to be sure, since they were often impossible to interpret. Indeed, the aims of doctors and patients were frequently at variance: the doctor's aim was negative urine tests while the patient's was to avoid hypoglycaemia, which could be achieved by keeping a little sugar in the urine.

Another area that was seriously deficient was patient education. In 1952 Beaser questioned 128 patients in Boston and found that all were 'distinctly deficient in knowledge of their disease'. Where the blame lay was unclear. He thought physicians often gave adults a half-hearted diagnosis ('a bit of sugar in the urine') and underplayed the potential seriousness of the disease.

In some countries continuing education involved admitting patients to hospital for a week for 'stabilization'. This was standard in Germany and Japan, even for changing the dose of insulin (which patients were forbidden to do). In England it was often used when someone was found to have a very high blood sugar in the clinic. Canny patients avoided this unwelcome

incarceration by omitting the meal before the clinic visit to produce an acceptably low result.

When insulin was introduced into clinical medicine, anyone
with a knowledge of human nature might have predicted that a
treatment that was under the patient's control would lead to trouble in some cases. Surprisingly, amid the general euphoria, problems of compliance do not seem to have been anticipated, possibly
because of the authoritarian Zeitgeist of the time, but more likely
because it was thought that those who had been saved from certain death would repay the discoverers of insulin by making the
most of their reprieve. In fact, faced with the seemingly impossible
task of keeping their urine sugar free, many patients simply gave
up or were crushed by conflicting priorities. Psychiatrists who
investigated patients with unstable diabetes often found that they
had chaotic and complicated private lives, which were invisible to
their physicians, who were, according to the psychiatrists, more
interested in treating the disease than the patient. One exception
was the Chicago physician Rollin T. Woodyatt (1878–1953), who is
credited with inventing the term 'brittle diabetes' for patients who
swung repeatedly from high to low blood sugar and were often
admitted to hospital with hypoglycaemia or ketoacidosis. In 1927
he wrote: 'I could give details of case after case in which the ups
and downs of the patients' tolerance were parallelled by events in
the psychic sphere.'[7] Most doctors treating diabetes did not take
much notice of psychological issues, but in 1944 two New York
paediatricians found that a third of children repeatedly admitted
with ketoacidosis came from broken homes, and many freely
admitted that they preferred hospital to home. One of the most
striking studies is one in 1949 by two psychiatrists in Baltimore,
who interviewed twelve adult patients, each of whom had had
over five admissions with ketoacidosis. Their doctors attributed

this instability to 'metabolic eccentricities', whereas all admitted to the psychiatrists that they had deliberately neglected or sabotaged their diabetic regimen. The same individuals disrupted their diabetes for different reason on different occasions, but, ultimately, all were trying to escape from stress by flight into hospital or by ending their own lives. Brittle diabetes, mainly in young women, has continued to be a difficult clinical problem to the present day and is often associated with an eating disorder. Such patients under-dose themselves with insulin so as to be able to eat as much as they want without gaining weight; thirst, urinary frequency, and vulval itching are the short-term price they pay.

Apart from the problems of kidney failure and blindness, another depressing feature of the diabetes scene after the Second World War was that the encouraging results in diabetic coma and pregnancy reported in the 1920s were proving difficult to replicate. For example, the mortality rate of diabetic coma in many large American hospitals was as high as 50 per cent. As usual the exception was the Joslin Clinic, where it was only 5 per cent. It was widely believed that this was due to a better class of patient and staff, but organization and facilities also played a part. At a nearby institution, the Massachusetts General Hospital (MGH), Boston, where the mortality was ten times higher, laboratory services were not available at night, weekends, or holidays. In 1944, 'after some chiding from Dr Joslin', ketoacidosis at MGH was treated as an acute medical emergency, so that a doctor was in constant attendance during the first twenty-four hours and a lab technician kept on duty until the patient was out of danger. This led to a dramatic drop in mortality.

Apart from the need for constant vigilance and attendance from the treating doctors, which was repeatedly stressed by Joslin, the management issues in treating ketoacidosis were:

should high or low doses of insulin be used? how should fluid be replaced? and, after 1950, should potassium be replaced, and if so, how?

High-dose insulin regimens became the norm after the Second World War as a result of authoritative reports from Howard Root (1890–1967) of the Joslin Clinic and John Malins in Birmingham. Root advised an initial dose of 100 units subcutaneously and 50 units intravenously, with a second dose half an hour later. It was anticipated that 200–300 units would be given in the first hour. Malins suggested that 200–400 units should be given at once intravenously, then 50 units every thirty minutes until the urine was free of acetone. Both Root and Malins produced tables showing reduced mortality on high doses of insulin, although both compared different time periods. For example, at the Joslin clinic a seventeen-year period before 1940 was compared to a four-year period after. Following these reports, large doses of insulin were recommended in most articles and textbooks for the next twenty-five years, but they were not universal. A low-dose regimen was started in Karlsburg, East Germany, in 1946 and continued for the next thirty years. Low-dose regimens were reintroduced in England and the rest of Europe from 1974 onwards as a result of the work of Peter Sönksen and have been universal since the mid 1980s.

In the 1940s it was not uncommon for patients with ketoacidosis to die hours or days after the start of treatment, when they seemed to be improving. Cardiac damage was usually blamed, but the explanation came from an American physician, Jacob Holler (1912–91). In 1946 he treated an 18-year-old who had developed ketoacidosis because she had not taken insulin for five days. After twelve hours of insulin and fluids, she had increasing difficulty breathing. Examination of the heart and lungs confirmed they were normal, but she could hardly breathe or move. Since she was obviously dying, she was put in an iron lung, a device used for patients whose respiratory muscles had been paralysed by polio. This was basically a large metal tank that enclosed the whole person apart from the head. After three hours of artificial respiration, Holler wondered if the paralysis was due to a low blood level of potassium (hypokalaemia). His hunch turned out to be right, and within twenty minutes of being given an infusion of potassium—a major logistical problem that involved opening the respirator and resuming artificial respiration—she was breathing normally. Hypokalaemia was almost certainly a common complication of the treatment of ketoacidosis, but for many years physicians were reluctant to give potassium, especially intravenously, because of a worry that it would cause cardiac arrest, as injections of potassium in animals did. The use of proactive intravenous potassium replacement was not generally accepted until the early 1970s.

Another area where results were suboptimal was pregnancy. In the late 1940s every other baby of a diabetic mother died either before or soon after delivery. Obstetricians were shocked by how quickly disaster could overtake a pregnancy that had seemed to be going well. In 1937 Raymond Titus (1883–1949) of Boston described a 21-year-old who developed ketoacidosis and labour at the same time and had a stillborn baby twelve hours later. Titus felt so badly about having lost a baby in front of his eyes, as it were, that he decided to deliver diabetic women by Caesarian section as soon as the baby was viable. He usually sterilized the women at the same time. A similar policy of early delivery was adopted at King's College Hospital, London, where in 1942 there were fifty-four pregnancies with an overall foetal mortality of 33 per cent. Women who had attended the diabetic clinic irregularly or not at all during pregnancy had a foetal mortality between 50 and 70 per cent and their babies typically weighed 9–10 lb (4–4.5 kg). Waiting for such a large baby to be delivered normally risked it dying suddenly in the womb or the shoulders getting stuck during labour. Delivery between the 36th and 38th week by Caesarean section seemed safer but introduced the dangers of pre maturity, especially if the woman's dates were wrong.

The only place where a perinatal mortality ten times greater than in the general population was not replicated was in Boston, where Priscilla White (1900–89) managed the diabetes. She had not finished her internship when Joslin recruited her in 1924. Her recollection was that, 'practically on my arrival, Dr Joslin assigned me to the study of diabetic children. He thought that, as the youngest member of the team, I would be close to them.' She also took over the medical management of diabetic pregnancies. She was intensely involved in the lives of her patients, to whom she wrote a letter after each and every visit. She was also greatly affected by foetal deaths, which may have been what pushed her towards aggressive management, particularly hormone replacement.[8] Her results in the 1930s were excellent, but in 1945 she introduced treatment with the female sex hormones, stilboestrol and progesterone; the results seemed miraculous. In women whose hormone levels were abnormal in early pregnancy, treatment increased survival of the babies from 54 to 89 per cent. Her clinical results were not replicated elsewhere, and in a UK Medical Research Council trial in 1955 the frequency of stillbirth and neonatal death was the same in hormone-treated and untreated women at 24–26 per cent. It was later shown that high doses of stilboestrol in pregnancy were harmful and caused cancer of the vagina in some offspring in their late teens or early 20s.

The most striking feature of infants of diabetic mothers was their large size (macrosomia), memorably described by the Scottish paediatrician Jim Farquhar (1922–98):

> The infants are remarkable not only because like foetal versions of Shadrach, Meshach and Abednego, they emerge at least alive from within the fiery metabolic furnace of diabetes mellitus, but because they resemble one another so closely that they might well be related...they convey a distinct impression of having had such a surfeit of both food and fluid pressed upon them by an insistent hostess that they desire only peace so that they may recover from their excesses.[9]

In 1952 a Danish physician Jørgen Pedersen (1914–78) proposed that high blood-sugar levels in the mother led to increased insulin secretion from the baby's pancreas and that this insulin acted as a growth hormone. His work first came to the attention of the Anglophone world in a paper in *Diabetes* in 1954. The 189 pregnancies he had managed between 1946 and 1953 were divided into two groups, according to when the woman was first seen—'long-term' patients were seen a minimum of fifty-three days before the expected date of delivery. The rest were 'short term'. The crux of management was an intensive effort to keep the blood sugar as nearly normal as possible, and it was measured four times a day in inpatients. This was successful in the long-term patients, whose mean in-hospital blood sugar was 7.4 mmol/l (133 mg/dl). Foetal mortality in the 111 short-term pregnancies was 36 per cent, and in the 78 long-term ones only 11 per cent. No hormone therapy was given, and the Caesarean section rate was only 8 per cent. Pedersen and the Professor of Obstetrics Ebbe Brandstrup updated their results in the *Lancet* in 1956. Between 1946 and 1955 they had managed 265 diabetic pregnancies and again divided them into long- and short-term groups. In practice women in the former group were admitted to the hospital on average sixty-five days before their due date, compared to thirty-five days for the latter. A single physician managed blood-sugar control in the hospital, and the average level achieved was 7.5 mmol/l (127 mg/dl). Foetal mortality in the long-term pregnancies was 8 per cent and in the short term ones 27 per cent. Comparing their results with those of Peel and Oakley in London and White in Boston, Pedersen identified the ingredients for success as (1) one attending physician and good medical treatment and (2) experienced obstetric and paediatric care by a few people. An equally important message was that it was unnecessary to do a lot of Caesarean sections or give sex hormones. Whether lengthy treatment in hospital was better than very close supervision as an outpatient (as practised by White) was impossible to say.

V

✹✹✹

TREATING LONG-TERM
COMPLICATIONS

As mentioned earlier, the tragedy of young diabetics with blindness or kidney failure was not publicized in the lay press, but dealing with these cases was a pressing problem for doctors in charge of diabetic clinics.

Eyes: retinopathy

In the 1950s the most serious form of retinopathy was (as it still is) the proliferative form in which fragile new blood vessels grow over the retina. Through the ophthalmoscope they look like fronds of seaweed, and, being unsupported, they are fragile and bleed into the jelly-like material (vitreous humour) inside the eye, causing either complete loss of vision or the sensation of looking through a spider's web. With luck the haemorrhage would be reabsorbed after a few days or weeks, with a return of normal vision. This reprieve might last a few weeks, but eventually there would be another bleed. It also might be reabsorbed, but eventually one would not clear, leaving the eye totally and permanently blind. By 1950 it had been established that the development of new vessels (neovascularization) was caused by a chemical or chemicals produced by a retina deprived of blood; this did not lead to any breakthrough in treatment until the 1990s, when one of these chemicals was identified as vascular endothelial growth factor (VEGF). Drugs that block VEGF have been developed, and it is hoped that they or related drugs may prevent proliferative retinopathy.

Back in the 1940s and 1950s oral drugs such as rutin (a glycoside from the rind of lemons that was supposed to strengthen blood vessels), vitamins C and K, and testosterone were tried, as was radiotherapy to the eye; all were ineffective, but continued to be used because there was nothing else to offer.

Faced with the rising tide of blindness in young diabetics, some doctors took desperate measures by removing the pituitary gland (hypophysectomy). The basis was a 1953 paper by a Danish physician, Jacob Poulsen (1907–88), 'The Houssay phenomenon in man: recovery from retinopathy in a case of diabetes with Simmond's disease'. Simmond's disease is atrophy of the anterior lobe of the pituitary gland (which produces growth hormone) as a result of uterine haemorrhage after childbirth. The Houssay phenomenon, discovered by the Argentinian Nobel prizewinner Bernardo Alberto Houssay (1887–1971), is a dramatic increase in insulin sensitivity after removal of the pituitary. In 1945 Poulsen's patient had a severe postpartum haemorrhage, after which her insulin dose fell from 80 units daily to 8 units every other day on which she had repeated severe hypoglycaemia. In the sixth month of pregnancy she had been noted to have (non-proliferative) retinopathy, but five years later this had disappeared. Poulsen wondered if the apparent cure of retinopathy might be a consequence of 'metabolic hormonal disorder' and suggested that removing the pituitary gland in young patients with severe retinopathy was worth trying.[1] This was first done in Sweden by the neurosurgeon Herbert Olivecrona (1891–1980) and the physician Rolf Luft (1914–2007). Luft was a friend of Poulsen and knew about the patient described above. Their first operation in 1951 was on a 30-year-old who was already blind in both eyes and had progressive kidney failure. It seems likely that the aim of the operation was to control his high blood pressure. Post-operatively his insulin dose dropped from 80 to 12 units/day, but he died of kidney failure. The next three patients were in their 20s and had the operation in an attempt to stop them becoming blind. The results were disastrous, with two dying on the day of operation and the other a month later. By 1955 Olivecrona had operated on twenty diabetics, of whom seven died within nineteen months of the operation. Some had improvement in vision and/or regression of new vessels, but the increased insulin sensitivity made their diabetes very brittle, and many died of hypoglycaemia. Critics pointed out the difficulty of selecting appropriate patients for what they called 'this mutilating operation', since, as they pointed out, retinopathy often waxed and waned and even new vessels could (rarely) regress spontaneously.

Hypophysectomies for retinopathy were never very common, and there was considerable doubt as to how effective they were. Nevertheless, they continued until the 1970s, when they were supplanted by photocoagulation (often called laser treatment). This was the brainchild of Gerd Meyer-Schwickerath (1921–92) of Essen, Germany. In 1946, after he had seen people with retinal burns from looking at the sun during an eclipse, he wondered if he would be able to stop new vessels bleeding by clotting them with heat. His first instrument used the sun as its light source, but, to make retinal burns, a fivefold magnification was needed, and, given the weather in Northern Europe, this was never going to be practicable. In 1949 he used a carbon arc lamp, which worked but was a nuisance, because it liberated sooty gases. He finally settled on a high-pressure xenon lamp, from which the spectrum of light emitted is similar to ordinary daylight.

Initially, Meyer-Schwickerath hoped to prevent bleeding from new vessels, but, because in many cases this was very frequent, treatment had to be repeated many times. A surprising finding was that, even in those who had received several hundred burns, the reduction of the visual field was remarkably small. Most eye specialists were sceptical about the value of light coagulation, and Meyer-Schwickerath thought that what eventually convinced them was 'before and after' retinal photographs, made possible by the invention in the 1950s of the electronic flash and the Zeiss retinal camera. In 1964 he published a paper on thirty-three patients he had treated in whom serial photographs showed a gradual diminution of hard exudates and macular oedema. An important observation was that new vessels often regressed *even if they had not been directly photocoagulated*. This was very important, because those that were most likely to bleed were the ones on the optic disc (where the optic nerve exits the eye), which could not be photocoagulated.

Adoption of light coagulation was relatively slow, because there was no absolute proof that it worked. 'Before and after' photos were all very well, but in many publications only the most dramatic ones were selected. There was also a suspicion that destroying the most alarming appearances of retinopathy was simply cosmetic. The xenon photocoagulator used by Meyer-Schwickerath needed up to 1.5 seconds to make the burn and was painful. The ruby laser introduced in 1960 had a pulse lasting less than half a second, was not painful, and was more easily controlled. There were many reports of uncontrolled studies in the late 1960s, but it was the enthusiasm of the respected Boston ophthalmologist William Beetham (1902–79) that convinced colleagues around the world of the value of laser treatment.

The driver of further research was a 1968 meeting organized by the United States Public Health Service at Airlie House, Virginia, where experts from all over the world were brought to discuss the problem of retinopathy and its treatment. Airlie House was a rural conference centre with no possibility of evening entertainment—except discussing diabetic eye disease! The original idea had come from two young doctors at the National Eye Institute, who suggested inviting the people who actually did the work rather than heads of department—a novel idea, since at the time funding to attend meetings was usually available only for heads. No individual papers were given, but participants were circulated beforehand with a proposed classification of retinopathy and in effect told to do their homework. A standard classification of retinopathy was crucial, because, in the absence of one, no conclusions could be drawn from over 1,200 hypophysectomies and 1,600 photocoagulations that had been done in the previous ten years. The leitmotiv of the meeting was the alarming increase in retinopathy and the lack of effective therapy, particularly for proliferative retinopathy. Participants agreed on the importance of randomized controlled trials, defined maculopathy, and decided on the importance of standard photos. Their work and collaborations dominated research and treatment of retinopathy for the next twenty years.

The American Diabetic Retinopathy Study (DRS) was planned as a direct result of the 1968 meeting and began in 1971. When the first report came out in 1976, it clearly showed that photocoagulation reduced the rate of severe visual loss in proliferative retinopathy. A year earlier preliminary results of a British trial showed that photocoagulation delayed the progression of maculopathy, the type of retinopathy most common in type 2 diabetes. The macula is the part of the retina used for sharp clear vision, such as in reading, and, when the blood vessels leak, as they do in diabetes, it leads to a build-up of fluid in the macula.

Photocoagulation was not a panacea but merely a way of stopping retinopathy getting worse. Even in the best hands there was still a 10 per cent or greater risk of progression of visual loss. It also had unavoidable side effects in the form of a reduction in visual field and night vision and, in the hands of careless or unlucky operators, excessive or misdirected burns, for example, on the macula.

Permanent blindness in people with proliferative retinopathy is caused by haemorrhage into the vitreous humour followed by scarring and retinal detachment. In 1972 a German eye surgeon Robert Machemer (b. 1933) made instruments with which it was possible to operate inside the eye. The vitreous humour could be sucked out and replaced with salt solution, bands of scar tissue could be cut, and detached retina stuck back on again. The technique was complex and the risk of complications high, especially in diabetic eyes. Nevertheless, a trial in 1985 showed that it was better than doing nothing. It is now widely used and leads to the return of useful, although never perfect, vision in people who have had massive haemorrhage in the eye.

Replacing the kidneys: dialysis and transplantation

Kidney failure (often referred to as uraemia) led to a particularly unpleasant death, with increasing anaemia and ill heath terminating in a phase of intolerable itching, vomiting, and breathlessness, which could last for weeks.

One of the main waste products excreted by a healthy kidney is urea from the breakdown of protein, and, since the beginning of the twentieth century, it had seemed logical to restrict dietary protein to treat kidney failure. This became standard practice in the 1960s in the form of the Giovanetti diet, named after its Italian inventor. It worked, but was rejected by many physicians, who believed that a high protein intake was essential for health and strength. There was a further problem for diabetic patients: when protein is severely restricted, calorie intake must be maintained to prevent loss of weight and muscle, which means filling the gap with carbohydrate. Diabetics who had been on a restricted carbohydrate diet for many years found it all but impossible to adjust to eating so much sweet stuff, and, in an age of technology, treating kidney failure with a machine was more attractive than diet.

An alterative to reducing the formation of urea was to remove it, and before the Second World War sporadic attempts were made to clean the blood artificially. The basis was dialysis, in which fluids with different concentrations of a dissolved substance are separated by a membrane through which small molecules can pass. Molecules from the high-concentration side diffuse through the membrane into the low-concentration side until the concentration is the same on both sides when movement stops. To treat kidney failure, blood was circulated through semi-permeable tubes in a fluid bath. Urea and other poisons that would normally be removed by the kidney were sucked out into the bath as the blood flowed through it. The person who made dialysis work was a Dutch physician, Willem Johann ('Pim') Kolff (1911–2009), who worked during the Second World War in the small town of Kampen. The membrane he used was cellophane tubing, which had been developed in the 1920s as an artificial sausage skin. The bath was made with the help of the manager of the local enamel factory. Between 1943 and 1945 Kolff dialysed sixteen people with kidney failure, and, although all showed temporary improvement, only one survived. Nevertheless, he showed that, in addition to fluid, various drugs and metabolites could be removed by dialysis. Amazingly under wartime conditions, Kolff built eight machines and later gave three to medical units in London, New York, and Montreal. Other physicians in the USA and Europe made dialysis machines, but the technical problems of running them were huge, and in 1965 Kolff guessed that half the 500 machines that had been made in the USA were gathering dust. At first dialysis was used only in acute renal failure to tide the patient over until kidney function returned. The breakthrough that permitted longer dialysis was made in 1960 by Belding Scribner (1921–2003), who devised a shunt that gave access to an artery. When Scribner first described the prolonged survival of patients with chronic renal failure treated by repeated haemodialysis, he was greeted with incredulity. It seemed unlikely that such a crude system could remove life-threatening impurities in the blood without depleting the patient of vital substances. A journalist described the process as 'surrendering one's life blood to a medical laundromat twice a week'. Chronic dialysis raised many ethical, moral, and economic questions. The first was whether the time bought would be worthwhile or simply a painful hanging on to life. There were undoubtedly cases in the latter category, but they were not publicized, and patients clamoured for the treatment, so that there was a gross mismatch between the available facilities and the number of potential patients. In the short term there was only one solution—selection of suitable patients and rejection of the rest. Candidates were often refused on non-medical criteria, so that they could be disqualified because of a previous history of criminality or antisocial behaviour. Kolff always emphasized the physician's duty not to judge. The first patient he treated in Holland in 1945 who survived was a 67-year-old woman who was admitted to hospital from a prison for collaborators and was not considered a useful member of society.

Diabetics with kidney failure almost always had other complications such as heart disease or retinopathy, and Kolff was one of the few physicians who did not automatically reject them. Unfortunately the results were dreadful. In a paper entitled 'The sad truth about haemodialysis in diabetic nephropathy', Kolff's group reported nine patients treated between 1967 and 1970; all were long-standing insulin-dependent diabetics with gross oedema. Three-quarters died during the first year, and depressingly there was no way of predicting the few who would survive for longer. The only glimmer of hope was that the longest survivor was a woman who had seemed initially to have the largest number of negative factors. Her three-year survival had, according to Kolff, been 'meaningful to her and her husband'.[2] In 1973, in response to the question 'What has regular haemodialysis to offer a 50-year-old hypertensive diabetic?', an expert in the BMJ suggested that dialysis was unlikely to offer an acceptable prolongation of life, commenting that 'the tragedy of a blind diabetic established on regular haemodialysis may result from unwise patient selection'.[3] Equally as discouraging as the high mortality was the poor quality of life of survivors. Most became blind, half developed such severe neuropathy that they could not walk without aids, and hardly any were rehabilitated to the extent of being able to go back to work. During the 1980s results gradually improved, although diabetics still fared badly. For example, in a 1988 report, just over half of type 1 and 2 diabetics on dialysis died in the first four years.

An alternative to dialysis was transplantation. The first successful kidney transplant between (non-diabetic) identical twins had been done in Boston in 1954. Tissue transplanted between identical twins is not rejected, and the long-term success of this case showed that kidney transplantation would work if rejection could be suppressed. The first immunosuppressant drug, azathioprine, became available in 1961, and with steroids it produced good results with live, related donors and greatly encouraged the development of transplantation. The 1970s ended with two important innovations, the use of tissue typing, which made rejection less likely, and the introduction of cyclosporine as an immunosuppressive agent.

In the 1960s the Minnesota transplant surgeon Richard Lillehei (1928–81) described uraemic diabetics as 'the pariahs of medicine'. According to him, diabetologists said, 'I can't take care of this patient, he/she has kidney failure,' and kidney specialists said, 'I can't take care of this patient, he/she has diabetes.'[4] Hence by 1972 only 19 of 5,432 kidney transplants worldwide had been done for diabetic renal disease, when diabetics would have been expected to make up 20 per cent of those eligible. Surgeons were reluctant to 'waste' kidneys on diabetic patients because of high death rates, fear that the combination of diabetes and immunosupression would lead to rampant infection, and the theoretical possibility of the new kidney being damaged by diabetes. The pioneers were at the University of Minnesota, where the first five diabetic cases from 1966 were combined kidney–pancreas transplants, the hope being that the pancreas would 'protect' the kidney by curing the diabetes. Unfortunately, the pancreas was usually rejected. Kidney transplants alone did not begin until 1968, but, by 1975, 132 operations had been done. Results were less good than in the non-diabetic, but much better than with dialysis. After three years only a quarter of diabetics on dialysis were alive, compared with more than half of those with a kidney transplant. By 1979 results in specialist centres in the USA and Europe had improved greatly, with two-thirds of patients still alive after four years and over 80 per cent of the kidneys still working. Transplantation and haemodialysis were restricted to younger patients. The middle-aged diabetics, originally described by Kimmelsteil and Wilson, did badly on haemodialysis, and there were not enough kidneys for them to have a transplant. A technique that was particularly suitable for them, continuous ambulatory peritoneal dialysis (CAPD), was introduced in the USA in 1976. It had been used occasionally in the previous twenty years, but only for short periods because of the danger of infection. Like other forms of dialysis, it works on the principle of osmosis, using the lining of the abdominal cavity (periotoneum) as the membrane between the dialysis fluid and the blood. A concentrated (hypertonic) solution is introduced into the peritoneal cavity, left for some hours, and then drained off, taking waste products such as urea with it. Advantages over haemodialysis in type 2 diabetics were that no access to an artery was needed and it avoided rapid shifts in fluid, which are particularly detrimental in heart disease, which many of these older patients had. Also, insulin could be added to the dialysis fluid, which was more physiological than giving it by injection, since it went straight to the liver. The major disadvantage of CAPD in general, and in diabetes in particular, was the risk of infection (peritonitis).

By the mid 1980s nearly a third of patients in the USA with end-stage renal failure had it on the basis of diabetes, most having type 2 diabetes. There was also a dramatic increase in the frequency of acceptance of type 2 diabetics for treatment of renal failure in Europe in 1985–90, although rates still remained half those in the USA. The method of dialysis varied from country to country. The preferred treatment in Germany and Austria was haemodialysis, and in the United Kingdom was CAPD.

Preventing or delaying kidney failure

High blood pressure was mentioned by Kimmelsteil and Wilson in the patients in their 1936 paper and was commonly found in young and old diabetic patients with kidney damage. From 1950 onwards several reasonably effective blood-pressure-lowering drugs were introduced, such as hydralazine (1951), methyldopa (1955), the thiazide diuretics (1958), and beta blockers (1960s), but diabetes specialists were not greatly interested in blood pressure. In the English textbook of Oakley, Pyke, and Taylor (1968), two pages were devoted to a discussion about whether hypertension was more common in diabetics than in the general population (surprisingly the answer was 'no'), and a half page to treatment. In the American textbook of Ellenberg and Rifkin (1970), high blood pressure merited only one paragraph. The main reason for disinterest in treating high blood pressure in general, and in diabetic kidney disease in particular, was a belief that reducing the pressure would reduce blood flow to the kidney and make matters worse.

In 1968 Malins had written in his textbook that 'there is no way of preventing or modifying the progression of nephropathy'.[5] The extraordinary change whereby within two decades reducing blood pressure became the cornerstone of treatment to stop diabetic kidney damage getting worse owed most to two Danish physicians, Carl Erik Mogensen (b. 1938) and Hans Henrik Parving (b. 1943), who worked independently. Mogensen's first study in 1976 was based on the observation that glomerular filtration rate (GFR), a measure of kidney function, worsened more rapidly the higher the blood pressure. The next stage was to see if reducing the pressure made any difference. Both Mogensen and Parving published studies in 1982–3 showing that effective blood-pressure lowering could more than halve the rate of decline of kidney function. These studies were criticized, because of the relatively small number of patients and the lack of a control group. Nevertheless, an important principle was established and has stood the test of time.

The question then arose as to how to detect the earliest stages of kidney damage. Mogensen's and Parving's index of kidney function was the glomerular filtration rate (GFR), which is too difficult to use in clinical practice. Proteinuria (protein in the urine) was the marker of nephropathy used in diabetic clinics, but available tests measured only relatively large quantities of protein, by which stage the kidney was already severely and irreversibly damaged. Luckily a test invented several years earlier was sitting, as it were, unused on the shelf. In 1963 Harry Keen (b. 1925) of Guy's Hospital, London, was looking for a way to document the earliest signs of kidney disease and wanted to measure small amounts of protein in the urine. With his research fellow he produced an immunoassay for albumin, which showed that many diabetics had small quantities of protein in their urine. They called this microalbuminuria—a misnomer, since what is being measured is not small albumin but small *quantities* of albumin. Surprisingly, microalbuminuria had already been discovered by the Ames Company. When they produced a tablet test for urine protein (Albutest) in the 1950s, clinicians complained that it gave 'false positives' in patients in whom the standard test for albumin was negative. In fact, Albutest was so sensitive that it was detecting microalbuminuria, but pressure from clinicians led to its replacement by a less-sensitive but more convenient dipstick, Albustix. By 1982 microalbuminuria was shown to be a marker of early nephropathy and later a more general indicator of bad blood vessels. It would become an important end point in trials of intensive treatment in diabetes.

Concurrently with research into microalbuminuria, a new class of drugs was introduced for hypertension, the angiotensin-converting enzyme (ACE) inhibitors. It was known from the early 1960s that ACE produced angiotensin II, which raised blood pressure. In the 1960s a Brazilian pharmacologist working in London found that a protein in Brazilian viper venom inhibited ACE, and his boss, the Nobel prize-winner John Vane (1927–2004), suggested that the Squibb company should try to make a synthetic ACE inhibitor. This was brave, since most experts did not believe that ACE had anything to do with ordinary symptomless (as opposed to the life-threatening malignant) hypertension. A chemist at the drug company Squibb did synthesize a nine-amino-acid compound (teprotide), which was effective but of no commercial interest, since it had to be injected and cost a million dollars per kilo to make. The project had effectively been scrapped, but in 1974 a biochemist, David Cushman, went back to the ACE inhibitor project, and within eighteen months had made captopril, which was launched in 1981 and became Squibb's first billion-dollar drug. More ACE inhibitors were subsequently made by other companies and have substantially improved the prognosis of type 2 diabetes by reducing the frequency of heart attacks and strokes.

Early detection of kidney damage and treatment with ACE inhibitors has led to a marked decrease in the frequency of end stage kidney failure. In the 1950s a third of type 1 diabetics developed kidney failure, whereas in the first decades of the twenty-first century less than 10 per cent of those with diabetes for thirty years have it.

Neuropathy

Diabetic nerve damage has always been a second-class complication in the minds of doctors and the public. It was not visible in the way that a white stick and guide dog are and, unlike kidney disease, did not cause death directly. The form that was of most concern to patients was painful neuropathy, but there was also a type in which the sensation of pain was lost from the feet and hands.

As mentioned in Chapter 1, Pavy had described the salient features of neuropathy in the nineteenth century, but medical interest waned until the publication of three large series of cases by William Jordan (1936) and Wayne Rundles (1945) in the USA and by Mencer Martin (1953) in London. Classification was difficult, because virtually every nerve in the body could be affected and the symptoms and signs were, in the words of Jordan, 'protean and may simulate many other diseases of the nervous system'.[6] Some patients had intense pain in the feet and legs, which began acutely but usually resolved within a few months. Others had an insidious onset of numbness, eventually resulting in the complete loss of sensation. In still others a single nerve was affected, resulting in double vision, facial paralysis, hoarseness, or foot drop.

It was by no means clear that nerve damage was due to diabetes per se. The three potential causes that were discussed in the 1950s and 1960s were atherosclerosis, vitamin deficiency, and disordered metabolism. Because neuropathy was at that time predominantly a disease of older patients, many clinicians thought that, like retinopathy, it was a senile degenerative change. Others, unable to explain neuropathy in young patients on the basis of atherosclerosis, separated the young and old and claimed that it was only in the latter that neuropathy was related to atherosclerosis, although this seemed unlikely, since hardening of the arteries without diabetes did not cause neuropathy. There was some similarity between diabetic neuropathy and nerve damage in dry beriberi, the condition caused by vitamin B1 deficiency. Many diabetic diets (especially those involving severe calorie restriction) were vitamin B deficient, and it was possible that B1, being water soluble, was lost in excessive amounts in the urine because of polyuria. Whether vitamins were beneficial in treating neuropathy was hotly debated, although they were widely used until the 1970s. Rundles pointed out that vitamin B supplements cured the neuropathy of beriberi in a few weeks but doubted whether they worked at all in diabetic neuropathy. He was sure that poor blood-glucose control was the cause of painful neuropathy and stressed that most of those affected had antecedent periods of months or years of poor control. In his view:

> Objective evidence of the lack of adequate diabetic care in patients developing diabetic neuropathy was seen in the nearly universal loss of considerable weight, not due to dietary restriction but usually with excessive food consumption, immediately before or during the period of development of the neuritic symptoms...94 of the 125 patients lost over 25 lbs of weight, 65 over 30 lbs and 40 over 40 lbs.[7]

Nearly thirty years later in the 1970s, the New York physician Max Ellenberg (1911–84) re-emphasized the extraordinary weight loss that might accompany acute diabetic neuropathy and suggested that it was part of a syndrome that he called 'diabetic neuropathic cachexia'. In six of his patients the loss of appetite and mental depression that accompanied the pain and weight loss had led to a provisional diagnosis of disseminated cancer. Another remarkable feature of this syndrome was that, even without specific treatment, all the (middle-aged or elderly) patients recovered spontaneously.[8] Rundles emphasized that diabetic neuropathy was an exceedingly painful condition, whose persistence over weeks and months tried even the most stoical personality. Where treatment was concerned, he recommended aspirin, supporting the bedclothes with a cradle, cool baths, and ice packs. Most experts recommended meticulous blood-glucose control, although some pointed out that sudden improvement of glucose control could actually precipitate painful neuropathy. It was also emphasized that the pain usually disappeared within a year or less. The pain of neuropathy was so bad that many doctors prescribed morphine, while others were strongly opposed to this, claiming that it would cause addiction. In the early 1970s treatment with the anti-epileptic drug epanutin (dilantin in the USA) or the antidepressant amytriptilene was shown to be moderately effective. Newer anti-epileptic drugs such as gabapentin have been shown to work better than epanutin with fewer side effects, but painful neuropathy remains very difficult to treat.

Painful neuropathy was always relatively uncommon and most diabetic patients with nerve damage had numbness or complete loss of sensation (anaesthesia) in their feet which was in the long run a much more serious problem as described in the next chapter.

VI

ADULT-ONSET DIABETES
AND TABLETS AT LAST

The debate described in Chapter 4 about whether good control prevented complications was understood to refer to those who developed diabetes in youth and were on insulin. They were greatly outnumbered by people who became diabetic after the age of 40, who until 1976 were called adult-onset or maturity-onset diabetics. They did get retinopathy and nephropathy, but their main problem was atherosclerosis. Two-thirds would die prematurely of heart attacks, and a striking finding was that women were equally affected; among non-diabetics heart attacks were four or five times more common in men, but in diabetes the sex ratio was equal. It was also clear that diabetes increased the severity of heart attacks, so that a first episode was more likely to be fatal or, if the person survived, to be followed by chronic heart failure. This knowledge did not have any practical consequences, because until the 1970s treatment for a heart attack was bed rest for five or six weeks, while nature took its course. Later, when heart bypass surgery was developed, it became clear that the reason why people with diabetes did so badly was that they had more extensive damage of the coronary arteries. Strokes were also more common in middle-aged diabetics, but, as with heart attacks, there was no treatment, and all that could be done was to wait and hope for natural recovery. The impact of adult-onset diabetes on public health was underestimated for many years, because, when a sufferer died of a heart attack, diabetes was omitted from the death certificate in more than half the cases.

The most feared complication was gangrene of the foot or leg, which was between twenty and fifty times more common than in the non-diabetic. Any black areas on the feet of diabetic patients were called gangrene, and in the 1930s, before the discovery of antibiotics, surgeons advised prompt operation before infection became established. They also favoured above-knee amputations, since these were most likely to heal. A justification for high amputations was the maxim that the diabetic's first amputation (on one limb) should be his last. This avoided the situation where the leg was removed in bits; a toe would be cut off and after a few weeks the amputation site would turn black. The foot would then be amputated through the ankle and again the wound would not heal. Eventually, after three or four operations, an above-knee amputation would finally heal. Early high amputation also made sense in people whose life expectancy was low—low because the hardening of the arteries that had caused gangrene in the leg was also present in the arteries of the heart, so that most died of heart attacks. In 1948 an American surgeon Samuel Silbert wrote that, 'by the time a diabetic has reached the point where he requires amputation of a leg for gangrene, his life has nearly run its course, and he will be among the select few if he is alive five years later. If alive, it is probable that loss of the second leg will have been necessary.'[1] In the 1930s nearly 50 per cent of diabetics having an amputation died in the immediate post-operative period. One reason for the high mortality was that inexperienced surgeons did these 'hopeless' operations. Another factor was that what Joslin called 'ward' patients (that is, charity rather than private patients) initially refused amputation and gave consent only when extensive gangrene and infection had set in. After the Second World War there was a big drop in post-operative mortality in most hospitals to around 10 per cent. This was attributed to antibiotics, although improved surgical techniques, better anaesthesia, and post-operative care, particularly the management of 'shock' learned during the war, played a part. Another factor that led to improved results was teamwork between physicians and surgeons. As Joslin put it, 'All the members of a [base] ball team cannot pitch the ball and no ball team wins which tries to have each member of the nine in the pitcher's box. It is only common sense to provide in a large general hospital for specialization in diabetic surgery.'[2] Common sense or not, diabetic surgery was not a speciality in most hospitals in America or Europe during the next fifty years.

A major economic problem was, and still is, the length of hospital stay and the time taken for rehabilitation. In the 1950s the average hospital stay after amputation was two months. In the 1990s it varied from country to country: sixteen days in the USA, twenty-eight in the UK, and forty-two in Holland.

In the 1940s, as an alternative to amputation, mechanical attempts were made to improve the circulation by putting the affected leg in a suction apparatus or placing the patient on an oscillating bed. Drugs that it was hoped would open up the blood vessels (vasodilators) included nicotinic acid, ganglion blockers, or, more pleasurably, whisky. Neither machines nor drugs worked. The obvious solution was to unblock the arteries or bypass the block, which was easier said than done. Bypassing an obstruction in the large femoral artery in the thigh with a vein was first done in 1949 and was fairly widely used by the 1960s. The long-term success in non-diabetics with a single block in the femoral artery was reasonably good, with more than half the bypasses still open after three years. Unfortunately, visualization of the arteries with angiography showed that most diabetics had multiple blocks in smaller arteries below the knee, where the results of surgery were poor. Even those who had only a single blocked artery were often denied surgery, because it was believed that the small vessels in the foot were diseased.

The use of antibacterial agents—sulfa drugs from the mid-1930s and penicillin, streptomycin, and chloramphenicol from the mid 1940s—made it clear that some diabetic foot lesions, especially in younger patients, were not due to arterial disease and would heal without surgical treatment provided infection was controlled. In England the recognition that neuropathy alone could cause gangrene owed much to the advocacy of Wilfrid Oakley (1906–98) of King's College Hospital, who in a lecture at the Royal College of Surgeons in 1954 introduced the idea of 'neurogenic gangrene'. He told his audience that loss of pain sensation was as important a cause of diabetic foot lesions as blocked arteries. These ideas were expounded to a wider audience in 1956 in the *BMJ*, where Oakley and colleagues wrote: 'It has been assumed too readily that [gangrenous lesions of the foot] are due to peripheral arterial disease alone or combined with a lowered resistance to staphylococcal infection. Careful examination of the great majority of these young patients shows that they have a quite adequate blood supply...the common defect being diabetic neuropathy.'[3]

Oakley focused on young patients, but neuropathic foot ulcers or 'neurogenic gangrene' could occur at any age. This type of ulcer

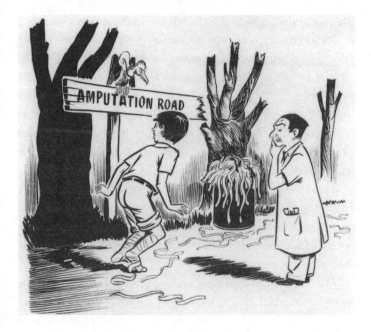

10. Paul Brand's 1966 warning that bandaging did not cure neuropathic ulcers in leprosy. (*Wellcome Library, London*)

was very familiar to doctors who treated leprosy, a disease that was mainly of interest to medical missionaries. One was Paul W. Brand (1914–2003), who, after working in India for twenty years, became chief of the Hansen's disease (leprosy) centre in Carville, Louisiana, in 1966. Since the nineteenth century, ulcers in people with insensitive feet had been called 'trophic ulcers', because they were thought to result from a lack of vitality in the tissues. Brand's contribution was to show that breakdown of the skin was due to repetitive (and painless, because of the nerve damage) pressure of a relatively moderate degree on the ball of the foot. Ulcers could also be caused by a stone in the shoe, which, because of the lack of pain, would literally burrow into the sole. According to Brand, results with leprous ulcers in India were very poor until 1939, when immobilization in a walking plaster became the standard treatment and led to relatively rapid healing. In a 1966 pamphlet for the Leprosy Mission, Brand wrote that 'the pathway to amputation of the leg is littered with bandages and dressings which have deceived both doctor and patient into thinking that by dressing an ulcer they were curing it...the whole problem is really one of mechanics not medicine'.[4]

Transmission of his message about the vulnerability of the anaesthetic foot to the world of (American) diabetes came about by chance. In the late 1970s Brand read an article about diabetic bone disease illustrated with x-rays that looked identical to the changes in the feet in leprosy.

He contacted the authors and was invited to address the Sugar Club, which he explained was 'a genteel group of diabetes specialists from the Southern states'. He described his work with leprous ulcers in India and his findings on repetitive stress. Most members of the audience were sceptical, pointing out that vascular disease was a complicating factor in diabetes but not in leprosy. However, John Davidson of Atlanta found that implementing Brand's ideas on minimizing pressure dramatically reduced the frequency of ulcers and amputations. Brand also opened the foot clinic at Carville to patients with diabetes and found that 'the notion of "non-healing wounds" proved as much a myth in diabetes as it had in leprosy. Our simple technique of keeping wounds in plaster casts for protection worked almost as well for diabetics. Ulcers chronic for years often healed within six weeks of the plaster cast routine.'[5]

Because of the vulnerability of diabetics' feet to ulceration, preventive foot care is now recognized as an important part of

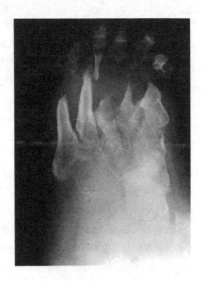

11. X-ray showing disintegration of the bones in a diabetic neuropathic foot. Similar appearances are seen in leprosy.

the treatment of a newly diagnosed middle-aged diabetic. As in so many other aspects of diabetes, Joslin was a pioneer in this. In the 1920s he set up a 'beauty parlour for diabetic feet' staffed by nurses whose mission was to teach the patient to 'keep his feet as clean as his face', because, in Joslin's words, 'it may seem a detail to tell the patients to wipe their feet gently, but if you wish them to avoid gangrene you must enter into these minutiae'.[6] For the next fifty years diabetes doctors paid lip service to the idea of preventive foot care, but in practice it was often neglected. It should have been the responsibility of chiropodists (called podiatrists in America), but in England before the Second World War they were few and usually ministered only to the middle and upper classes. Chiropody was not mentioned in the 1948 National Health Service Act, and for the next thirty years hospital chiropodists in England were part-time, poorly paid, and restricted in the scope of what they could or were allowed to do. They were basically 'padders and parers', whose main allegiance was to orthopaedic surgery. Joslin had a chiropodist as part of his team from 1928 onwards, and in 1936 Harold Himsworth (1905–93) asked the founder of the Chelsea School of Chiropody to provide a service at University College Hospital, London. Himsworth explained that 'care of the feet of diabetics was a great problem, since gangrene and perforating ulcers were the nightmare of the physician'. Joan Walker (1902–95) in Leicester appointed a chiropodist as part of her team in the early 1950s and credited him and antibiotics with having reduced the frequency of gangrene. However, provision for chiropody to diabetic clinics in England remained patchy. Diabetes foot clinics are now common, the first having been established at King's College Hospital in 1981, with the dramatic result that the amputation rate was halved by 1986. Nevertheless, there are many areas and countries where amputation rates remain shockingly high, with gross disparities between the best and worst.

Treating adult-onset diabetes

From the end of the nineteenth century onwards the 'great men' of diabetes stressed the importance of patient education and diet as the linchpins of treatment. What varied greatly was how conscientiously individual physicians organized and audited educational programmes. Whether instruction should be given in a class or in some other form varied from country to country and probably depended on the size of the hospital. Classes were popular in the USA and Germany, but in England teaching was usually done one to one by ward sisters, dieticians, and chiropodists. Unfortunately the teachers, although well meaning, had not been taught how to teach, and their lessons were often overly scientific and perceived by the recipients as being completely negative—don't do this, don't eat that. The author of a 1920 article about diabetes education commented: 'There is no use in talking in the language of the laboratory to a patient who understands only the language of the kitchen. We must either teach him the new language or translate our Greek into understandable English.'[7] Unfortunately this was ignored in diabetic units for the next sixty years. In a survey of British diabetic clinics in 1975, 12 per cent used posters for dietary education, 15 per cent food models, and 8 per cent group teaching, while 59 per cent advised the spouse. A fifth did not use any aids but relied on instruction given by the doctor and sometimes the dietician or health visitor. Surveys showed that physicians prescribed an amazing variety of diets, most of which were not adhered to. In Sweden in 1942–3, 53 per cent of people with a diabetic ration card said they were not following their diet very carefully and 10 per cent were not following it at all. In 1948, in Leeds, England, dietary adherence was described (by the physician) as 'hopeless' in a third of patients, while in 47 per cent it was 'tolerably satisfactory'. A 1967 American survey found that only one in eight patients was even approximately following his or her prescribed diet. The failure of dietary treatment to result either in permanent weight loss or in control of diabetes was usually blamed on the ignorance or disobedience of patients, but most physicians knew little about nutrition or diet, and did not seem to realize how difficult it is to change eating habits. In a talk to the American Dietetic Association in 1961, a psychoanalyst pointed out that, if the patient was a furnace that passively accepted any diet offered, there would not be a problem. However, he continued, 'the patient is anything but passive and will only take a diet of foods which are available and afford-able, satisfy his taste and his aesthetic values, are culturally and socially acceptable, and can be served in amounts and at times that fit into his own routine and that of his family and social group'.[8] He further put the boot in by suggesting that healthy middle-class American physicians and dieticians assumed that their preferences for food, patterns of eating, and appetites were shared by mankind in general.

When diet failed to reduce blood-sugar levels enough, the only other treatment until the 1950s was insulin, which was started reluctantly in overweight middle-aged people, because it caused weight gain and worked less well than in younger peo-ple, so that large doses were often needed. The work of Wilhelm Falta (1875–1950) in Vienna and Himsworth in London had established the principle of insulin sensitivity and resistance. Basically, young thin people (who would now be called type 1 diabetics) responded to a small injection of insulin with a large drop in blood sugar, they were prone to hypoglycaemia, and, when deprived of insulin, their blood sugars rose rapidly and they developed ketoacidosis. Older fatter people (type 2 diabet-ics) needed many more units of insulin to cause an equivalent fall of blood sugar, and even large doses did not cause hypoglycae-mia. Stopping insulin for twenty-four hours led to only a mod-est rise in blood sugar, and they did not develop ketoacidosis.

In 1951 insulin in the blood was measured for the first time in humans by the Polish-born Australian physician Joseph Bornstein (1918–94). He did this by injecting the patient's serum into a rat in which sensitivity to insulin had been increased by removing the pituitary and adrenal glands. Working with Lawrence in London, Bornstein found that no insulin was detectable in five people with newly diagnosed juvenile diabetes, while five overweight adult-onset diabetics all had measurable levels. This confirmed the paradigm that young diabetics had insulin deficiency, while in older patients there was insulin but something was interfering with its action. One candidate was growth hormone from the pituitary gland, since people with acromegaly (where a tumour overproduces growth hormone) often had insulin-resistant diabetes. This idea gained favour when, in 1937, the biochemist Frank Young (1908–88) found that injections of pituitary extract caused permanent diabetes in cats and dogs and later showed that this was due to growth hormone. Another possible culprit was overactivity of the adrenal gland, since many middle-aged diabetics, especially women, were red faced and hairy, like people with Cushing's syndrome (overactivity of the adrenal cortex). Cortisone, the main hormone produced by the adrenal cortex, was first used as a drug in 1949 and had miraculous effects in rheumatoid arthritis. Patients who had been bed- or wheelchair-bound walked again, but large doses were often needed, so that many developed diabetes as well as high blood pressure and stomach ulcers. Some synthetic drugs also caused diabetes. The thiazide diuretics (still widely used in the treatment of high blood pressure) were introduced at the end of the 1950s, and it soon became clear that they were diabetogenic, especially in people with a strong family history of the disease. In 1962 a related compound, diazoxide, was found to cause acute reversible diabetes in almost everyone who took it. It continued to be used occasionally for the next thirty-five years as a treatment for insulin-producing tumours of the pancreas (insulinomas). Another drug that could cause or precipitate diabetes was the oral contraceptive pill first marketed in 1963. During the next decade a huge and confusing literature built up on its alleged diabetogenic effect. Some suggested that what the pill did was to unmask latent diabetes in women who were assumed to have a 'poor pancreatic reserve', on the basis of a family history of diabetes or a history of large babies. The early pills contained large doses of oestrogen and worries about precipitating diabetes largely disappeared with the introduction of low-oestrogen and progesterone-only pills in the 1970s.

Tablet treatment for diabetes

The discovery of insulin stimulated a search for orally active compounds to lower blood sugar. In the 1920s Collip thought that, because plants contained glycogen, they would have an insulin-like hormone. He made extracts from yeast, onion tips, lettuce, sprouted grains of barley, and even lawn grass, which did seem to lower the blood sugar of rabbits. Collip proposed the name 'glucokinin' for the active ingredient of these extracts, but his results were never confirmed.

The perennial herb *Galega officianalis*, also known as goat's rue, had been used as a folk remedy for diabetes since the Middle Ages. The active ingredient was found to be a chemical called guanidine, and attempts were made to modify the guanidine molecule to increase its blood-sugar-lowering action and make it less toxic. The result was synthalin, which in 1926 Minkowski hailed as something 'that could help the great army of mild and medium severe diabetics'. Unfortunately it caused loss of appetite, nausea, diarrhoea, and, most seriously, liver damage. Samples were sent to the British Medical Research Council, but it was unimpressed, and the drug was withdrawn in England in 1928. In May 1927 the highly respected Carl von Noorden published an account of an oral pancreatic preparation that was said to have been obtained by 'strong tryptic digestion of fresh pancreas substance'. It was given the name 'glukhorment' and attracted a lot of attention. The Horment company sent samples to Henry Dale at the National Institute for Medical Research in London, but when analysed it was found to contain synthalin. A similar conclusion was reached independently in Prague. When he heard these results, von Noorden considered the only two explanations—that synthalin had somehow been synthesized during the process of production process, or that it had been dishonestly added. The latter was obviously more likely and foreshadowed scandals in the 1990s, when 'natural diabetes cures' turned out to be laced with glucose-lowering drugs such as glibenclamide (see below).

The discovery of drugs that could stimulate the pancreas to produce more insulin was serendipitous. In 1942 Marcel Janbon, a physician in Montpellier in the south of France, used a new sulphonamide antibacterial agent to treat patients with typhoid. Some had fits or became unconscious and were found to have hypoglycaemia. A physiologist, August Loubatières (1912–77), tested the drug in dogs and found that it caused severe hypoglycaemia. It had no effect in depancreatized animals, and he therefore suggested that it must increase insulin release from the pancreas. It still worked in animals with only 10 per cent of the pancreas left, and Loubatières thought it might be useful in diabetes, provided there were still some working islet cells. This work, published in French, went unnoticed for many years.

Carbutamide, the first of the class of anti-diabetic tablets called sulphonylureas to be marketed, was synthesized in 1945 in Dresden as an antibacterial agent. In 1950 it was used in (Communist) East Germany to treat urinary infections but found to cause hypoglycaemia, and their ministry of health banned it.

The head of research at the company that had made carbutamide moved to West Germany, where he joined the drug company Boehringer Mannheim, which arranged for the drug to be tried on diabetic patients in Berlin. Like synthalin 30 years earlier, it reduced blood sugar, but only in adults who had had diabetes for less than ten years and had not used insulin for more than 1–2 years—that is, people who still had some insulin reserve. The results were published in a prominent German medical journal in 1955 and aroused great interest worldwide among diabetics and their doctors. In 1956 issues of the *Canadian Medical Association Journal* and the *BMJ* were devoted to the new drug. The *BMJ* took a holier-than-thou approach, claiming that diet was ignored in most of the German patients, so that far more were on insulin than would have been the case in a British clinic, where 'they would be dieted without insulin'. The idea that a drug could increase insulin secretion was treated with scepticism. Writing in the *BMJ*, the prominent biochemist Frank Young noted that most drugs that lowered blood sugar were also anti-microbial and wondered (wrongly, as it turned out) if they worked by killing insulin-degrading bacteria in the liver.

One reason for caution about the new drugs was concern about side effects. Sulphonamides, which are related to sulphonylureas, had been used against infections for more than ten years, and even short courses could cause serious allergic reactions and fatal bone-marrow damage. Diet was already a safe remedy for mild diabetes, and—so the argument went—any alternative must be equally innocuous. Carbutamide was tested in America by Eli Lilly, but side effects occurred in one in twenty patients, and there were several deaths. The problem of its toxicity was summed up by the Eli Lilly's research director, who wrote:

Actually the toxicity of carbutamide is comparatively quite low. Certainly it would be no deterrent to treatment of any serious temporary illness, e.g. pneumonia, nor would it be considered serious if no other safe treatment were available for diabetes. It is a nice question to contemplate—how much toxicity can be tolerated in a drug used in the management of a disease which may extend over an ordinary lifetime?[9]

The effectiveness of carbutamide stimulated a search for safer drugs. The first was tolbutamide, made in 1956 in the Hoechst laboratories in Germany. Like carbutamide, it worked best in older, fat patients with short-duration diabetes. It was thought to work by stimulating beta cells to produce more insulin, but there was concern that it might eventually exhaust them to the point where insulin injections would be needed. A second sulphonylurea, chlorpropamide, was introduced in 1958 and was more potent and longer acting.

An editorial in the journal *Diabetes* pointed out the well-known improvement of blood-sugar control simply by seeing patients more often, and remarked that tablets worked best in those who did not need them—overweight adults with mild diabetes. The editorialist thought it deplorable that newspapers had created the false hope that diabetes was now easy to control because tablets were available. It was a common perception of diabetes specialists that the new drugs might encourage slackness in diet. Also they worried that, while they lowered blood sugar, the drugs might not have any effect on diabetic complications.

Two guanidine compounds (biguanides) that worked in a different way from the sulphonylureas were introduced at the end of the 1950s. One was phenformin, the usefulness of which was limited by side effects of nausea, diarrhoea, and a metallic taste in the mouth. How it worked was uncertain, but there was a suspicion that, like synthalin, it poisoned the liver. It was eventually withdrawn in the 1980s because of a high frequency of deaths from lactic acidosis. The possibility of serious side effects was a big worry to doctors. The idea that drugs could be harmful had been brought dramatically into the public domain in 1961 by the thalidomide scandal, in which a drug that had been promoted as a safe remedy for morning sickness in pregnancy was found to cause serious birth defects.

The other guanidine compound was a drug that had been discovered in 1929 but forgotten. In 1956 a French clinical pharmacologist Jean Sterne (1909–97) joined a small pharmaceutical company whose boss asked him to look into the claim that the forgotten drug was useful in influenza. After preliminary animal experiments, Sterne found the drug lowered blood sugar in humans. It was introduced as metformin at the 1958 International Diabetes Federation Conference, but was received unenthusiastically. Its real value was not recognized until the 1990s, and it has since become a mainstay of the treatment of type 2 diabetes.

By 1960, 500 scientific papers had been published on the sulphonylureas and biguanides. Yet, there were many unanswered questions. (1) In whom should they be used? (2) What about side effects? (3) Would they prevent diabetic complications? (4) Were they better than insulin?

It was clear that tablets, alone or in combination, could not replace insulin in young patients. However, many older patients could be weaned off insulin onto chlorpropamide, a longer-acting sulphonylurea than tolbutamide, or a combination of chlorpropamide and phenformin.

The idea persisted that sulphonylureas might wear out the pancreas. Indeed, they often failed to control blood sugar after working for months or years (called secondary failure). Some of these failures may have been due to disregard of diet but most were due to progression of the disease as a result of declining pancreatic function. The only way of establishing the value of the new drugs was to compare them to the gold standard of insulin, and this led to a highly contentious clinical trial.

The University Group Diabetes Program

This attempt to find out whether oral hypoglycaemic agents prevented diabetic complications began in 1960 when some American academic clinicians and a statistician met to plan what became known as the University Group Diabetes Program (UGDP). They wanted to find out if blood-sugar-lowering treatments prevented or delayed complications and to study the natural history of vascular disease in adult-onset diabetes.

Patients recruited were those in whom diabetes had been diagnosed less than a year earlier and who, in the opinion of their physicians, were likely to live at least five years (the length of the original funding). The study began in 1961 with allocation to one of four regimens:

1. *Insulin variable*: as much insulin as necessary to maintain normal blood glucose.

2. *Insulin standard*: a fixed dose of Lente once daily according to the patient's surface area. This group was included to distinguish between the blood-sugar-lowering and other possible effects of insulin.

3. *Tolbutamide*: a fixed dose of 1 gram before breakfast and 0.5 gram before the evening meal, chosen because it was the average dose used in clinical practice.

4. *Placebo*: Lactose tablets or capsules.

In 1962 a fixed-dose phenformin group was added.

It was hoped to recruit 200 patients in each group, but this proved so difficult in the twelve university clinics that special screening procedures were used to find new diabetics. No attempt was made to exclude patients with vascular disease, and it later transpired that patients in one centre were recruited from the cardiac clinic. It was, of course, expected that the mortality would be lower in the insulin and tolbutamide groups than in those on diet alone. However, the tolbutamide arm of the study was stopped prematurely in 1969, because analysis by what the *Lancet* called 'advanced, elaborate, and novel statistical techniques' showed a significantly higher death rate in the tolbutamide group (12.7 per cent) than in the placebo group (4.9 per cent). Mortality in the two insulin-treated groups was nearly the same as for placebo patients. In 1970 an ad hoc committee of the American Diabetes Association commented that, apart from the apparent toxic effect of tolbutamide:

> What is even more arresting is that neither of the insulin-treated groups had a lower mortality than the placebo-treated patients. This finding carries the broadest implications for the treatment of non-insulin-dependent adult onset diabetes. First, if insulin—the diabetic's medicinal remedy sine qua non—does not permit patients to live longer than does a diet, would not this class of patients, in respect to longevity, be just as well off with diet alone? Secondly, if insulin can do no better with mortality than diet, is it likely that any oral hypoglycemic agent presently available, whether or not it acts by stimulating insulin secretion, can do any better than the hormone itself or even as well?[10]

These findings, together with work (discussed in Chapter 8) by Marvin Siperstein (1925–97) suggesting that complications were genetically determined, implied that most forms of treatment in adult-onset diabetes were a waste of time.

To say that the findings of the UGDP did not go unchallenged would be a major understatement. In 1975 the *Lancet*'s summary was: 'The storm of controversy aroused by these results is probably without parallel in modern medicine. Every aspect of the trial has been minutely criticized by clinicians and statisticians, while supporters of the trial have defended it with equal vigour.'[11]

The US Food and Drugs Administration (FDA) endorsed the conclusions and announced that warning labels would be put on all oral anti-diabetic drugs, whereupon forty leading American diabetologists who had not been involved in the UGDP trial hired a lawyer to prevent the FDA proceeding with its labelling proposal.

Arguments about the study were both personal and scientific and were fuelled by what opponents saw as the self-righteous tone of some UGDP spokesmen. An example of personal animus was the revelation that the statistician Christian Klimt had been a paid consultant to the manufacturers of phenformin. Supporters countered by claiming that their opponents were 'drug company whores' paid by the makers of tolbutamide, which had been so tarnished by the study.

The most cogent scientific criticisms were summarized by Holbrooke Seltzer of Dallas, Texas, in the journal *Diabetes* in 1972 and rebutted by the UGDP investigators in an article in the same journal.

According to critics, the odds were stacked against tolbutamide from the start, because factors favouring cardiac death such as angina and abnormal ECGs were commoner in the tolbutamide group. They believed the randomization had broken down, although the differences could easily have arisen by chance. The investigators countered that their critics seemed not to appreciate the purpose and power of randomization. This may have been true, since the FDA demanded randomized controlled trials for the first time in 1962, and this was the first in diabetes. Before 1962 the evidence in support of therapeutic efficacy put to the FDA was often just 'testimonials' from physicians who casually tested experimental drugs on their patients and were paid for doing so.

One critic, James Moss of Washington, commented that 'there were 30 deaths in the tolbutamide treated patients with 20 in each of the other groups. Never before have 10 deaths created such a controversy.'[12] He pointed out that 50 per cent of the tolbutamide patients who died had autopsies, compared to only 29 per cent of those on placebo or insulin. If only three deaths in each group had been reassigned, the statistical significance of the increased cardiovascular deaths in the tolbutamide group would have disappeared.

Deaths were unevenly distributed between clinics, so that, as one would expect, the three that enrolled the sickest patients had most fatalities, and the three that admitted the healthiest had least. Moss wrote sarcastically that 'the one thing this study proves is that patients who already have heart disease die sooner than those who do not'. The English physician Arnold Bloom (1915–92), a master of the *bon mot*, used to say that in some centres swallowing tolbutamide was like drinking cyanide, while in others it was as innocuous as eating sweets.

Most patients came from underpriviledged groups where compliance was known to be a problem and only 26 per cent remained on their assigned treatment for the whole study

The credibility of the conclusion that insulin was ineffective in reducing cardiovascular deaths was greatly weakened, since almost half of those on variable insulin who died of cardiovascular causes had had virtually no insulin.

When the critics finally got the records under the Freedom of Information Act in 1971, they found evidence of sloppy data recording and mismanagement. Just over half of those studied had a fasting blood glucose under 130 mg/dl (7.2 mmol/l) at baseline, leading Moss to ask how it was possible to evaluate the benefit of a drug that lowers blood-glucose levels, if only 46 per cent of the patients actually had hyperglycaemia.

How much effect the UGDP had on clinical practice is hard to say. My impression is that American doctors were sharply polarized. In the early 1970s a friend of mine worked in an American clinic where oral agents were banned. Patients who failed on diet were put onto insulin, with the dose being increased 'until the syringe had been filled'. Then the patient was left, in the words of Arnold Bloom, 'to stew in their own sugar'. At the other end of the spectrum, Joslin Clinic doctors ignored the UGDP, noting in 1971 that oral agents had been used in 10,000 of their patients for as long as ten years and that they were 'here to stay for the foreseeable future'. The UGDP findings were heavily criticized by European opinion leaders and medical journals. No official warnings were issued, and sulphonylureas and biguanides continued to be used by the 30–40 per cent of patients in an average European clinic who were on tablets.

By the beginning of the 1970s it seemed to many that the treatment of adult-onset diabetes was a mess. But several important scientific advances had been made in the previous fifteen years that laid the basis for future therapeutic progress.

VII

AT THE LABORATORY BENCH

I n the 1950s many countries including England, Germany, the USA, the Netherlands, and Canada had indigenous manufacturing industries producing the two most popular modified insulins, NPH and Lente. Most doctors thought these were satisfactory, and in 1954 a well-known American specialist begged the manufacturers to be cautious about adding more 'to the present ample market'. No doctor asked for purer insulin preparations, but purification was the goal of insulin chemists, and became the Danish manufacturers' trump card in increasing their market share.

In the 1920s and 1930s minor allergic reactions at the site of injections (such as itchy lumps) were quite common. With increased purification they became rare, and it was clear that allergy was due to contaminants rather than to insulin itself. In contrast to the rarity of allergy, unsightly cosmetic effects at injection sites were common. Lipoatrophy, where the subcutaneous fat at an injection site melts away, was so common that in most clinics in the 1940s and 1950s half the patients (especially women) had at least one patch. It was eventually found to be caused by insulin antibodies (see below). Fatty lumps at

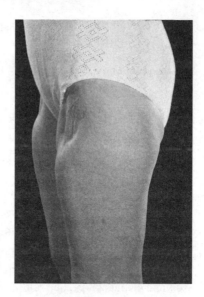

12. Area of lipoatrophy at the top of the thigh where insulin injections have caused the fat to melt away.

injection sites (lipohypertrophy) were due to direct stimulation of fat production by insulin and were commonest in children, who discovered that injecting into them was relatively painless.

That insulin was an antigen, or something that stimulated the production of antibodies, became the basis of a method for measuring insulin in the blood. The delicate bioassay in animals used by Bornstein (and others) was supplanted in the early 1950s by test-tube methods in which a patient's serum was added to rat diaphragm or testicular fat, and glucose uptake or glycogen synthesis was measured. These lacked specificity, because other substances in the blood could produce insulin-like effects. Between 1956 and 1960 an exquisitely sensitive and specific method, the radioimmunoassay, was developed by Solomon Berson (1919–72) and Rosalyn Yalow (b. 1921). Berson, a physician whose research skills were self-taught, met Yalow, a physics PhD, in New York in 1947. Berson had not trained in endocrinology and why they became interested in insulin is not clear. Possibly it was because Yalow's husband was an insulin-dependent diabetic, although her biographer suggests that the stimulus was a 1952 paper in which Arthur Mirsky (1907–74), uniquely both a biochemist and a psychoanalyst, hypothesized that type 2 diabetes was due to abnormally rapid degradation of insulin by a hypothetical enzyme that he called insulinase. If this was right, insulin would disappear from the circulation faster in type 2 than in type 1 diabetics or normal subjects. Berson and Yalow combined insulin with radioactive iodine, so as to be able to measure it with a Geiger counter. It was then injected into normal subjects, diabetic patients, and one schizophrenic having insulin coma treatment. Contrary to Mirsky's hypothesis, insulin disappeared rapidly in normal subjects and diabetics who had not been treated with insulin. In diabetics who had been on insulin for more than a few weeks and in the schizophrenic who had had scores of injections, it disappeared much more slowly. To investigate this they invented a way of separating plasma proteins and found that, in the serum of people treated with insulin, the radioactivity migrated with gamma globulins—the protein class that forms antibodies. They deduced that insulin was attached to anti-insulin antibodies. This was contrary to received wisdom that small proteins like insulin could not be antigenic (provoke the formation of antibodies). When Berson and Yalow sent their paper to the elite *Journal of Clinical Investigation* (*JCI*) in 1956, the editors were so offended by the idea that insulin might be antigenic that they agreed to publication only if the words 'insulin-transporting antibody' were removed from the title. The editor-in-chief told them that the expert reviewers emphatically rejected their 'inescapable conclusion' that the insulin-binding protein was an antibody. Nevertheless, within a few months their findings were confirmed by others, and the *JCI* published their next paper, 'Ethanol fractionation of plasma and electrophoretic identification of insulin binding antibodies', without a whimper.

During the next few years Berson and Yalow studied insulin from a variety of animals and, *inter alia*, found that the antibodies formed when pork insulin that was injected into guinea pigs reacted very strongly with human insulin. This led them to devise the radioimmunoassay, a technique for measuring minute quantities of any substance to which an antibody can be produced. They first used their new assay to measure the concentration of insulin in humans, and the results were published in 1960. Among their early findings was that fat people with type 2 diabetes had high insulin levels, whereas more severe diabetes was associated with insulin deficiency. Berson died in 1972, and, since Nobel prizes cannot be awarded posthumously, Yalow was awarded it alone in 1977. In her acceptance speech, Yalow, who attracted adjectives such as 'arrogant', 'belligerent', and 'overbearing', pointed out that immunoassay had been slow to take off, and included a slide showing that until 1965 virtually all the papers on it in prominent journals were by her and Berson. Within a decade the technique had been extended to virtually all other hormones and is now used to diagnose and monitor almost every endocrine disease. The striking exception is diabetes, which is still defined by blood-glucose levels rather than by the amount of the hormone in the blood.

Prelude to synthetic insulins

In 1925 the American pharmacologist John Jacob Abel (1857–1938) crystallized insulin and found that in chemical tests it reacted as a protein. Most scientists dismissed the idea that proteins could have specific biological properties, but, by 1938, when a German chemist Hans Jensen wrote a 250-page monograph on insulin, it was clear that insulin was a protein. According to Jensen, its activity depended on the whole molecule and on how the component building blocks (amino acids) were linked. This jigsaw was solved by a Cambridge biochemist, Fred Sanger (b. 1918). Apart from the fact that it was biologically important, Sanger chose insulin because its chemical composition had been studied extensively. Seventeen different amino acids had been identified in beef insulin (the type most commonly used in treatment). It was known to contain a lot of the sulphur-containing amino acid cystine, and the integrity of the bonds between cystine molecules was considered essential for its activity. These disulphide bonds are important in maintaining the 3D structure of proteins. Sanger started his research in 1943, but after six years working alone had discovered the sequences of only two short substructures. At this rate the full sequence of the fifty-one amino acids would have taken another half century. Luckily in 1949 he was joined by the Austrian Hans Tuppy, and three years later they had elucidated the whole structure. Sanger had always assumed that the molecular weight of insulin was 12,000, but in 1952 it was shown to be 6,000. He worked out that it consisted of two chains with three disulphide bonds and not four chains, as he had originally thought. In 1955 Sanger published the full structure, bringing to a close what was described as the major venture of modern biochemistry. In *The Times* Sanger's achievement was described as the biochemical equivalent of running the four-minute mile, a feat achieved by Dr (later Sir) Roger Bannister in Oxford a year earlier. Sanger was awarded the 1958 Nobel Prize for chemistry, and in 1980 won a second for determining the nucleotide sequences in DNA.

Knowing the amino-acid composition of insulin was important, but to know how it worked on a molecular level it was essential to know the 3D structure or how the chains were arranged in space. This was worked out in Oxford by Dorothy Hodgkin (1910–94) using X-ray crystallography. The idea that X-rays might be used to unravel the structure of a crystal by working back from the angles of reflection and intensities of the reflected rays was developed by William Bragg, and his son, Lawrence, in Cambridge before and during the First World War. Hodgkin remembered a sentence from William Bragg's book for schoolchildren that read: 'the discovery of X-rays has increased the keenness of our vision over ten thousand times and we can now "see" the individual atoms and molecules.' She worked first on penicillin, which had only thirty-nine atoms. Her next project was vitamin B_{12}, with over a thousand. It took Hodgkin and an army of helpers eight years to solve its structure, for which she was awarded the 1964 Nobel Prize for chemistry.

Her interest in insulin began in 1935 when she put a crystal in front of an X-ray beam with a photographic plate behind it. That night, when she developed it, she saw minute, regularly arranged spots forming a pattern of reflections from the individual atoms. She was so excited that she roamed the streets of Oxford dreaming that she might be the first to know the structure of a protein. She never imagined that it would take until 1969 for her to work out the structure of insulin.

Even before the 3D structure of insulin had been worked out, it had been made from scratch in a test tube. An important stimulus was the finding in 1960 that, when the A and B chains were disconnected, its activity was lost, but was regained by recombining them. Therefore, in theory the chains could be made separately and then put together. This was first done by Panayotis Katsoyannis in Pittsburgh in 1963. It was followed almost immediately by the synthesis and combination of A and B chains of sheep insulin by Helmut Zahn (1916–2004) and co-workers. Surprisingly this feat was achieved in the German Wool Textile Research Institute where Zahn was the director. The skill that he learned in his wool research was a knowledge of cross-linking agents, which was important for wool processing and finishing. In 1965 the complete insulin molecule was synthesized from amino acids by Wang Ying-lai (1908–2001) and colleagues, in Shanghai, China. Insulin thus became the first protein of any type—as well as the first human protein—to be made chemically. However, the process was extremely laborious, and it was clear that it could never be commercially viable.

For several years after the structure of insulin had been established, it was unclear how it was made in the body; the A and B chains might be made separately and then joined, or they might be formed as a single chain and then split. In 1967 Donald Steiner (b. 1930) of Chicago showed that it was made as a single-chain precursor with a molecular weight of 9,000. He called the precursor proinsulin and showed that it consisted of the A and B chains joined by a connecting or C-peptide. It was found that patients with insulin-producing tumours had a large proportion (30–85 per cent) of proinsulin in their circulation, and this has been a useful diagnostic test to distinguish between insulinomas and hypoglycaemia caused by surreptitious injections of insulin (as in murders by insulin). Since one molecule of C-peptide is produced for every molecule of insulin, measuring C-peptide made it possible to measure endogenous insulin secretion in patients who were on (animal) insulin and had anti-bodies that interfered with the immunoassay.

Berson and Yalow had shown that insulin caused the formation of anti-insulin antibodies, but how much this mattered in clinical practice was debatable. Certainly, antibodies could interfere with the action of insulin—cases of patients on 6,000 units of insulin a day (as opposed to the usual 40–60) were spectacular but very rare. Most patients with high titres of antibodies needed only slightly higher doses of insulin than those without. There was a positive side to antibodies in that they prolonged the action of soluble insulin and had a 'smoothing' effect, so that patients with antibodies (as most of them had until the 1960s) managed well on two injections of soluble insulin per day. There was even a suggestion that *lack* of antibodies might result in greater swings of blood sugar and 'brittleness'. Studies that suggested this beneficial effect were not published until the mid 1970s, and, by this time, the tail had already wagged the dog in the direction of as little antigenicity as possible.

Originally antibodies were thought to be an inevitable consequence of injections of a foreign protein, with beef insulin being more antigenic than pork because it differs from human insulin by three amino acids whereas pork differs by only one. However, during his research on proinsulin, Steiner found that insulins made from animal pancreata could be split into three distinct peaks by a technique called gel filtration. Peak A contained large pancreatic proteins, B was proinsulin and related materials, while C contained mainly insulin. A team at the Novo research institute in Copenhagen found that peaks A and B had a powerful effect in promoting antibody formation when injected into rabbits. They managed to purify pork insulin, so that the concentration of contaminants was reduced from 1,000 parts per million to less than

20. Such purified insulins did not cause antibody formation and were marketed in 1973 under the trademark 'Monocomponent' (MC). Novo's Danish competitor Nordisk followed suit with RI (rarely immunogenic) insulins. These preparations usually led to a modest reduction in insulin dose, but their most dramatic, albeit cosmetic, effect was to prevent lipoatrophy. Until 1980, when Novo and Nordisk gained a foothold, Eli Lilly and Squibb dominated the market for insulin in the USA. Most Lilly insulins were 70 per cent beef and 30 per cent pork, while Squibb's, although not labelled as such, were pork for short-acting and beef for long-acting. In the early 1970s both Lilly and Squibb improved the purity of their insulins from a proinsulin content of 10–40,000 parts per million (ppm) to 300–3,000 ppm. Lilly called insulin of the latter degree of purity 'single peak'.

There was a belief (especially in the Novo company) that insulin antibodies played a part in the development of retinopathy and nephropathy, although they could not be *the cause*, since diabetics who had never been on insulin also got these complications. A major factor (apart from advertising) pushing clinicians into using the new highly purified insulins was a 1976 paper by Stephen Bloom and colleagues in London emotively entitled 'Dirty insulin: a stimulus to autoimmunity'. Bloom found that British-made beef insulins contained significant amounts of glucagon and other pancreatic hormones, whereas highly purified Danish pork insulins were free of them. The introduction of highly purified insulins brought about a fundamental change in the insulin market. Previously physicians had regarded insulin as a generic product like petrol. In other words, if the chemist had run out of Boots insulin, the Wellcome or Weddel equivalent would be just as good. The new Danish insulins had trade names associating them with a particular producer—Novo's Actrapid was particularly memorable. New and old insulins were not interchangeable, so that, for example, replacing Boots beef-soluble insulin with highly purified pork Actrapid led to major changes in glucose control. Novo and Nordisk reps had always eulogized the purity of their insulins, and Bloom's paper added a scientific reason for switching from the old 'dirty' insulins. Novo and Nordisk began a campaign to 'educate' European doctors by inviting opinion leaders to symposia in Copenhagen—lesser doctors had to manage with meetings in their local area.

The Danish insulin manufacturers did not invent new insulin regimens, but they played a major part in their commercial success. In the 1960s, most physicians in Europe and the USA put their patients on either one daily injection of PZI (70 per cent) or a twice-daily mixture of soluble and isophane (30 per cent). A few, such as Francis Lukens (1899–1978) of Philadelphia, thought that insulin regimens should attempt to mimic the way insulin was produced in the body—peaks coinciding with meals and a low level during the night. In 1965 he suggested that this could be reproduced only by injections of quick-acting insulin before each meal. He also suggested that soluble or regular insulin in some way protected against complications regardless of variations in blood sugar. In Europe, multiple injections of soluble insulin were used in 1968 as part of a research project by the Paris physician Georges Tchobroutsky (b. 1930). His aim was to see if better glucose control, which it was assumed would be obtained with multiple injections, reduced the rate of progression of retinopathy—they seemed to do so slightly, although the number of patients was too small for definite conclusions. Multiple injections were regarded as experimental, and it is difficult to say what the typical insulin regimen was in the 1970s. Probably, as with views on control, it varied from country to country and clinic to clinic. Michael Berger (1944–2002) told me that when he came back to Germany from the USA in 1978, 90 per cent of German diabetics were on once-daily surfen insulin. When I worked at King's College Hospital, London, in the early 1970s, most patients were on one daily injection of PZI or twice-daily soluble and isophane. The exceptions were 'old stagers' diagnosed in the 1930s, who had stayed on soluble insulin for up to forty years. By the late 1970s in England the regimen of twice-daily soluble and isophane had increased in popularity. The problem was that, when isophane (which lasts 8–12 hours) was given with the evening meal, it peaked too early, causing hypoglycaemia around 3 a.m., and then ran out, leading to hyperglycaemia before breakfast. Increasing the dose to overcome this simply resulted in worse hypoglycaemia during the night. The solution was a 'peakless' long-acting insulin such as bovine Ultratard, which after five or six days built up to produce constant basal insulin levels, especially at night. It worked quite well with bovine Ultratard (as a similar scheme had twenty years earlier with PZI), but, when pork and later human Ultratard replaced the bovine product, the very long action was lost and the regimen was no better than twice-daily soluble and isophane.

What caused multiple injections to take off was the invention in 1981 of the insulin pen (Penject) by the Glasgow physician John Ireland (1933–88), who, as befits an inventor, was as much at home under the bonnet of a car as at the bedside. Injections had become more convenient after the introduction of plastic syringes in the 1970s, but Ireland's device combined the syringe and vial of insulin in a single unit in which one simply dialled up the dose. The original was rather cumbersome, but the idea was taken on board by the Novo company, which in 1985 launched

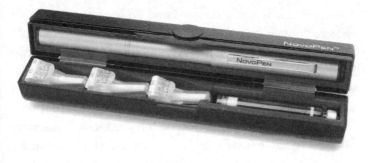

13. Novopen, a device for giving insulin injections. (*Novo-Nordisk, Copenhagen*)

NovoPen®, a sleek metallic device that won design awards as well as being very popular with patients. The NovoPen was part of a package of multiple injections, and, although it gave them a competitive advantage, Novo promoted the so-called basal–bolus regimen of an injection of Actrapid before each meal with long-acting insulin in the evening. Such regimens had always seemed to many doctors to be 'physiological', but few patients could be persuaded to take a syringe and insulin vial to work with them. Insulin pens changed this.

Human insulin

In 1974 a team at the drug company Ciba Geigy produced human insulin by total synthesis. The process was expensive, and only enough for a short-term study in six diabetics and three patients with insulin allergy was produced. The results were not particularly startling, but there was a feeling that human insulin must, in some vague and unspecified way, be better for human diabetes than material derived from animals. Hence, to produce it became the holy grail of pharmaceutical companies, in spite of the fact that highly purified pork insulins had already eliminated lipoatrophy, allergy, and insulin resistance. The driving force was commercial, in that it was thought that, faced with a choice between human and animal insulins, customers would unhesitatingly choose the former. The first human insulin, the result of collaboration between the Genentech and Eli Lilly companies in the USA, was produced by genetic engineering in 1981. The human insulin gene was inserted into the E. Coli bacterium, which, after growing in a culture medium, produced insulin. The Novo Company soon did the same thing with yeast—in effect brewing insulin. The US Food and Drugs Adminstration, which was notorious for its tardiness in approving new drugs, took only five months to review and approve Lilly's Humulin. Whether this haste was due to enthusiasm for the first product of genetic engineering or whether it owed something to a potential shortage of animal pancreata is uncertain.

Biosynthetic human insulin was a great scientific achievement, but the practical benefits were rather underwhelming, and in blind trials neither the investigators nor the subjects could distinguish between pork and human insulin. Nevertheless, Eli Lilly and Novo were desperate for human insulin to succeed to justify their investment and to free themselves from the abattoir, with its theoretical risk of contaminating insulin with prions such as bovine spongiform encephalopathy (BSE). The result was an advertising campaign (to doctors) promoting the benefits of human insulin, which was described as 'identical to the body's own insulin and therefore the logical choice' (Novo) or 'outstandingly pure and less immunogenic than that which comes from the pancreas of pigs or cattle' (Eli Lilly). Marketing was so successful that between 1984 and 1988 more than 80 per cent of patients in the UK had been switched to human insulin, which cost twice as much as the products it replaced. The switch was often made autocratically by doctors, who justified it by claiming that the 'old-fashioned animal insulins' were about to be withdrawn, as had been suggested (unofficially) by drug company representatives.

Some patients who were changed to human insulin were dissatisfied and in particular complained that their warning symptoms of hypoglycaemia differed or were lost completely. There was also a suggestion in the late 1980s that human insulin was responsible for young diabetics who were found dead in the morning in an undisturbed bed having been normal the previous evening; this so called dead-in-bed syndrome had been reported before, but it seemed to be more common with human insulin. In fact the deaths were almost certainly due to hypoglycaemia and unrelated to the species of insulin.

If asked what innovation had made the most difference to their lives in the 1980s, type 1 diabetics in England would unhesitatingly have chosen not human insulin but the spread of diabetes specialist nurses.

Diabetes specialist nurses (DSNs)

In the 1930s Joslin proposed 'wandering diabetic nurses' to help general practitioners. He claimed that they would save the doctor's time and also teach patients to use insulin and diet and 'combat coma and gangrene'. Like many of Joslin's initiatives, this fell on deaf ears, but was implemented in England by Joan Walker in the 1950s. The job description made it clear that her DSNs were to be nurse, dietician, chiropodist, social worker, psychologist, and detective rolled into one. Their main job was education, which had to be 'slow, painstaking and above all consistent'. Another of Walker's innovations was treating newly diagnosed children at home. The justification was that 'there is much less disturbance in the child's life when everything seems to be against him'.[1] It did, of course, disturb the lives of hospital-based paediatricians and did not become common practice in England for over thirty years.

When I went to Nottingham in 1975, there were less than ten DSNs in the UK, but numbers gradually increased, so that by 1990 there were over 400 and by 2008 most clinics had three or four. The idea was also taken up during the 1980s in North America, where DSNs are called diabetes educators. Whatever their title, these people (mainly women) did more in the last two decades of the twenthieth century to improve the standard of diabetes care than any other innovation or drug. Above all they have humanized the service and given the patient a say in the otherwise unequal relationship with all-powerful doctors. The success of DSNs in diabetes has stimulated other disciplines to appoint specialist nurses for other chronic conditions, such as asthma or inflammatory bowel disease.

Using technology to treat or cure type 1 diabetes

People with type 1 diabetes were usually excited by the prospect of new insulins, only to be disappointed to find how little difference they made to their lives. Managing diabetes was still a chore that needed relentless attention, 24 hours a day for 365 days a year—what someone described to me as 'a lifetime without holidays'.

For those who already had the disease, the desideratum was a cure, while those who, because of their family history, worried that their children would become diabetic, hoped for some means of prevention. In the 1980s and 1990s, both seemed tantalizingly just over the horizon.

Those who already had type 1 diabetes hoped for something that would manage diabetes without any effort or dietary restriction on their part—an artificial pancreas or a transplant of insulin-producing cells.

The first attempt to mechanize control of blood glucose was made in 1964 by Arnold Kadish of Los Angeles. His device, which was carried on the back and weighed several kilos, worked, and he made the important observation that 'very small amounts of insulin administered on a continuous basis intravenously are more effective than much larger doses administered as usual [subcutaneously]'. In the 1970s machines were made that incorporated a sensor to measure blood glucose, a computer-controller to process the results, and a pump to infuse insulin or glucose into a vein according to an algorithm or mathematical prescription. One was the Biostator made by Miles Laboratories, which worked, although its disadvantages far outweighed its advantages. It was expensive (about $55,000 in 1982), the patient was confined to bed or a chair, and the machine needed constant supervision to recalibrate the glucose-measuring device and respond to (frequent) alarms and malfunctions. It was suggested (apparently seriously) that the Biostator could manage a hospital patient 'over the weekend', but this was a complete fantasy. The reality was that most machines purchased were relegated to cupboards within a year or two.

In the 1970s it was thought that glucose-sensing and insulin-delivery problems could be solved quickly by intensive application of existing technology, but that information handling would remain problematic, because it needed so much computing power. In practice, the opposite turned out to be the case; computer technology advanced exponentially, but no continuous glucose sensor had been produced by the beginning of the twenty-first century.

More practical than the Biostator was a system described in 1974 by Gérard Slama and associates from Paris. A pump was carried in a shoulder bag and delivered insulin intravenously. It worked quite well but was limited by the need for constant intravenous access. Nevertheless it showed what could be done and led directly to continuous subcutaneous insulin infusion (CSII), first used in 1978 by John Pickup and Harry Keen at Guy's Hospital, London. They used the Mill Hill pump, a relatively small battery-operated device that delivered small pulses of insulin through a needle under the skin every few minutes to replicate the constant low level of background insulin in people without diabetes. Larger pulses were given thirty minutes before meals. Using CSII, some people achieved better control than with conventional injections, although much of this may have been due to extra attention to their diabetes. Pickup's paper was followed by a rash of publications reporting highly satisfactory results in *selected* patients—I stress the word selected, because pumps were not a panacea for poor glucose control; they required much attention from the user, and, because there was no depot of insulin, interruption from kinking or blockage of the tube led to ketoacidosis. By 2008 pumps had been reduced to the size of a pager and have elaborate programmes for the basal rate of insulin infusion and premeal boluses. The main advantage cited by users is increased flexibility of lifestyle, and the main disadvantage cost—about £2,500 for a sophisticated pump and £1,000 per year for consumables. In

2000 it was estimated that there were over 200,000 pump-users worldwide, more than half of whom were in the USA.

Pancreas transplantation offered a potential cure of type 1 diabetes. The first was done in 1966, when Richard Lillehei transplanted a kidney and pancreas in a 28-year-old woman, who died three months later after many complications. Worldwide in the next eleven years, fifty-seven transplants were done, but only two worked for more than a year. Mortality was high, and there were many surgical problems; the main difficulty was dealing with the corrosive enzymes secreted by the exocrine pancreas. The major innovation in the 1970s was to block the pancreatic duct with glue so that the enzyme-producing tissue withered—a repeat of Banting and Best's work.

There was a passionate debate about the justification for pancreas transplantation. Unlike heart or liver transplants, where the recipient would die without one, there was an alternative for the diabetic—to continue on insulin injections. On the other hand, for the patient a successful operation meant insulin independence and freedom from dietary restrictions and hypoglycaemia. It is easy to see why people who already had kidney failure might be prepared to take the extra risk entailed by a combined kidney–pancreas transplant.

An attractive alternative was to transplant the islets alone. The leader in this was Paul Lacy (1924–2005) of St Louis, who in 1967 isolated intact islets from rat pancreas and had moderate success in 'curing' diabetes by transplanting them in inbred rats, which, like identical twins, do not need immunosuppression. In both rats and people, islets are transplanted by injecting them into the portal vein; when they reach the liver, they lodge in smaller branches of the vein. In the 1980s and 1990s it always seemed that the problem of islet cell transplantation was about to be solved, but by 1999 only 8 percent of 267 recipients were totally free of insulin injections one year later. Hope was rekindled in 2000 by the much-publicized work of a team in Edmonton, Canada. After five years, 80 per cent of their transplanted patients were producing some insulin, but only 10 per cent could manage without any injected insulin. Edmonton patients were given about 20 per cent of the normal number of islets, and even this requires up to four pancreata, which could have been used as whole organ transplants for four patients with a much better long-term success rate. It seems inescapable that islet cell transplantation will not be possible on a large scale unless human islets can be grown from stem cells. Alternatively, pig islets could be used, and either 'humanized' or encapsulated to protect them from the recipient's immune system.

Like the artificial pancreas and islet cell transplantation, prevention of type 1 diabetes has always seemed on the verge of being achieved since the 1980s. The reason for optimism is that it is an autoimmune disease in which antibodies generated in the body attack an organ. Also it can be identified before all the insulin-producing cells have been irreversibly damaged. In the early 1900s several pathologists noted that the islets of some young people who had died of diabetes were infiltrated by lymphocytes (insulitis). This was forgotten until 1965, when a Belgian pathologist, Willy Gepts (1922–91), found it in fifteen of twenty-two young diabetics who had died within six months of the onset of the disease, but not in those who had died after having diabetes for more than a year. The number of beta cells was reduced, and those that remained were bigger than normal, as if, Gepts thought, they were desperately attempting to produce insulin. Presciently, he remarked that 'it seems probable that in the pancreas of acute diabetics [those who died within six months] we had the opportunity to catch the final stages of a process which has been going on for an indefinite time, perhaps from birth'.[2] One of Gepts's subjects also had lymphocytic infiltration of the thyroid gland, and he suggested that the infiltrates in the islets and thyroid might be due to the newly discovered pathological process called autoimmunity. He was referring to the discovery by Deborah Doniach (1912–2004) of the Middlesex Hospital, London, of antibodies that destroyed the thyroid gland, causing myxoedema, and others that attacked parietal cells in the stomach, causing pernicious anaemia. Another glandular disease with lymphocytic infiltration was (non-tuberculous) Addison's disease, and again the blood contained antibodies against the adrenal gland. By the late 1960s it was clear that glandular diseases involving autoantibodies and lymphocytic infiltration—Addison's, myxoedema, and pernicious anaemia—were more common in people with type 1 diabetes but not in those with type 2. It therefore seemed likely that type 1 was caused by autoantibodies against the islets. In the event, islet cell autoantibodies (ICA) were not discovered until 1974. The main reason for the delay was that, unlike those in thyroid and adrenal disease, which persist indefinitely, ICA disappear in most people with type 1 diabetes during the year after diagnosis.

The (apparently) acute clinical onset of type 1 diabetes and the fact that it more commonly started in the winter had long suggested an infectious cause. One possibility was mumps, which had been known since the nineteenth century to cause pancreatitis and rarely to be followed by diabetes. However, since most children had mumps and very few children became diabetic, it was obvious that the relationship could not be very strong. In the late 1960s interest in an infection was rekindled by the finding of higher titres of antibodies to the Coxsackie B4 virus in newly diagnosed diabetic children. However, further epidemiological studies gave inconsistent results, and attempts to make mice diabetic by infecting them with viruses were generally unsuccessful.

In 1972 the study of identical twins mentioned in the Prologue showed that fewer than half the pairs were concordant (both affected) for type 1 diabetes, which suggested that an environmental factor must be involved. Epidemiology supports this idea. For all the attention it gained as a result of the discovery of insulin, diabetes in the young was uncommon in the first half of the twentieth century, but during the second half the incidence rose by about 3 per cent per year in most Western countries and North America. There was also an extraordinary variation in incidence between countries from 3/100,000 per year in Macedonia to 54/100,000 per year in Finland. In Estonia, which is less than 100 kilometres away, the incidence was only a third of that in Finland.

During the second half of the twentieth century childhood type 1 diabetes rose in parallel with that of asthma and predominantly affected affluent people in temperate climates. This strongly suggests an environmental factor, and among those suggested have been lack of breast feeding (or early exposure to cow's milk), inoculations, or early weaning. Alternatively, it is possible that modern living in the West has removed a protective factor—dirt. A rodent that develops autoimmune diabetes, the NOD (non obese diabetic) mouse, does so much more often if reared from birth in a sterile environment. The hygiene hypothesis suggests that for both humans and the NOD mouse the immune system needs to be challenged by infections and other environmental factors to develop properly. Failure to do so, so the hypothesis goes, results in autoimmunity or allergy (for example, asthma). What particular infection or infestation might have been protective is speculative, but one that has been suggested is the pinworm (sometimes called threadworm), an intestinal parasite that causes anal itching and was once carried by a large proportion of children, but is now very much rarer.

The discovery of islet cell antibodies and the association of what was called juvenile-onset or insulin-dependent diabetes with specific tissue (HLA) types indicated that it and diabetes in older people (called maturity-onset or non-insulin-dependent diabetes) were separate diseases. In recognition of this, in 1976 Andrew Cudworth (1939–82) renamed them type 1 and 2 diabetes, and this terminology is still used. Classifying diabetes on the basis of the age of onset or the type of treatment had always been unsatisfactory and became more so when it was found that 5–10 per cent of older people with apparent type 2 diabetes had islet cell antibodies and that most of them needed insulin sooner rather than later. It is now clear that they have late-onset type 1 diabetes, which is now called LADA or latent autoimmune diabetes of adults. An unexpected finding from the Barts Windsor Study of the epidemiology of diabetes in children, started by Cudworth, was that ICA could be detected in siblings of young diabetics up to ten years before the siblings developed apparently acute onset diabetes. This did not completely rule out the possibility that a virus had originally triggered the process, but did show that there was a long lead-in period during which intervention might prevent continuing beta-cell destruction. The hope had always been that a specific viral infection would be identified as the trigger for type 1 diabetes, since inoculation against the virus would prevent it. Even without knowing the trigger, there was hope that the autoimmune process could be stopped. Studies to this end were undertaken in patients with newly diagnosed diabetes using the anti-rejection drug cyclosporin (1986) and in relatives at high risk of developing diabetes with the vitamin nicotinamide (2004) and even small doses of insulin (2002), but none was successful. These failures are particularly frustrating, because, in the best animal model of type 1 diabetes, the NOD mouse, over 100 different interventions can prevent diabetes.

VIII

∞∞

THE PHARMACEUTICAL ERA

I have called this chapter 'the pharmaceutical era', because after 1980 treatment of diabetes came to be dominated by increasingly powerful drug companies. Between 1960 and 1980 no new insulins or drugs had been introduced, and the pharmaceutical industry seemed disinterested in diabetes. However, an increasing target population, especially in the USA, the largest and most profitable market, made them keen for a slice of the action. They also came to realize that they could set the agenda by advertising to, or ingratiating themselves with, prescribers. The concept of drug companies targeting opinion leaders was not new but became increasingly important in the last two decades of the twentieth century.

Forming a society of interested doctors is an important step in establishing a speciality such as diabetology—a term first used in America in the 1980s. The American Diabetes Association (ADA) was formed in 1941, the International Diabetes Federation (IDF) in 1952, the medical and scientific section of the British Diabetic Association in 1959, and the European Association for the Study of Diabetes (EASD) in 1965. By the end of the twentieth century meetings of these organizations were so large that only a limited number of cities had the facilities to host them. For example, the 2007 meeting of the ADA in Chicago had 13,000 attendees and that of the IDF in Cape Town 12,700; in fact, diabetes is the poor relative. Meetings of cardiologists and gastroenterologists are even larger. Drug companies pay much of the cost of these meetings, and the content is always in danger of being tainted by what one critic called 'gaudy commercialism'. One factor that undoubtedly energized doctors and drug companies to take a renewed interest in diabetes was resolution of the control complications debate. After the UGDP study many doctors, especially in the USA, had a nihilistic view of the value of diabetes treatment. They agreed that relieving symptoms was worthwhile but contended that nothing would prevent long-term complications. Apart from the UGDP findings, their main evidence was a paper in the influential *Journal of Clinical Investigation* in 1968 by Marvin Siperstein, who studied specimens from the main thigh muscle, the quadriceps, under a microscope and claimed that 90 per cent of adult diabetics and 50 per cent of 'pre-diabetics' (children of two diabetic parents) had thickened capillary blood vessels. He used the quadriceps because it was easily accessible and he assumed that the findings in muscle blood vessels reflected what was happening to small blood vessels in the eyes, kidneys, and nerves. Improbably he found that thickening did not increase with the duration of diabetes, whereas clinical studies always showed that, the longer someone had had diabetes, the more microvascular complications (retinopathy, nephropathy, and neuropathy) there were. He also claimed that basement membrane thickening did not occur in non-genetic diabetes, such as that following pancreatitis. Siperstein concluded that retinopathy, nephropathy, and neuropathy were genetically determined and hence unpreventable. His views, although eventually discredited, were remarkably influential, and in 1976 a group of doctors from the ADA attempted to squash the heresy that blood-glucose control was unimportant. In an editorial in the *New England Journal of Medicine* they laid out the (circumstantial) evidence that good glucose control prevented complications and stated that treatment should include 'a serious effort to achieve levels of blood glucose as close to those in the non diabetic state as feasible, particularly in those at greatest risk of microvascular complications, the young and middle aged'.[1] Doctors dislike being dictated to, and other prominent specialists (including Siperstein) produced a counter editorial suggesting that aiming for normal blood sugars was impractical and that any benefit would be offset by serious hypoglycaemia. Both groups were taken to task by the editor, who pointed out that the debate was marred by hazy definitions and a lack of facts. The implication was that a proper trial was needed, and this led to an American trial in type 1 and a British one in type 2 diabetes.

Neither would have been possible without two advances in the late 1970s, self-monitoring of blood glucose (SMBG) and haemoglobin A1c (HbA1c). The former allowed people on insulin to feel safe with sugar-free urine tests and the latter provided an objective measure of glucose control.

From the 1950s, measuring blood glucose in the laboratory became easier and more accurate. The Technicon AutoAnalyzer (1957) could make hundreds of measurements in a day, and using the enzyme glucose oxidase instead of copper reagents made the test specific for glucose. The disadvantage was that results were not available in real time, because blood had to be taken from a vein and transported to the lab, and then the result sent back to the doctor. The first 'instant' blood-sugar method was the 1964 invention at Miles Laboratories, Indiana, of a test (dextrostick) in which a large drop of blood was taken from a fingerprick, put on a paper strip impregnated with chemicals, and washed off after sixty seconds. The deeper the blue colour that developed, the higher the glucose concentration. In 1970, the Ames reflectance meter was made to 'read' the stick. An American engineer, Richard Bernstein, asked Miles if he could buy one. They refused to sell to patients, but he got one through his wife, who was a doctor. By measuring his blood sugar five times a day (and taking a very low-carbohydrate diet) he managed to put his diabetes in order. He later qualified as a doctor and has been a zealous advocate of the need for people with diabetes to take control of their own disease. In 1968 a German firm Boehringer Mannheim introduced a strip from which the blood was wiped rather than washed. They also marketed a meter, the reflomat, which, like the Ames meter, was large, mains operated, and needed careful standardization.

That these meters might be used by patients was not considered until 1975, when Dr Clara Lowy of St Thomas's Hospital, London, suggested that a 26-week-pregnant woman who was finding it difficult to control her diabetes should be admitted for regular monitoring. After a few days in hospital the woman insisted that, if loaned a meter, she could do the tests at home, which she did for the rest of her pregnancy. Some of Lowy's colleagues and many other doctors considered this irresponsible and dangerous. However, she and colleagues at St Thomas' Hospital and a group in Nottingham published papers in 1978 showing that ordinary people could measure their own blood sugars. Those who took part liked SMBG, which helped them

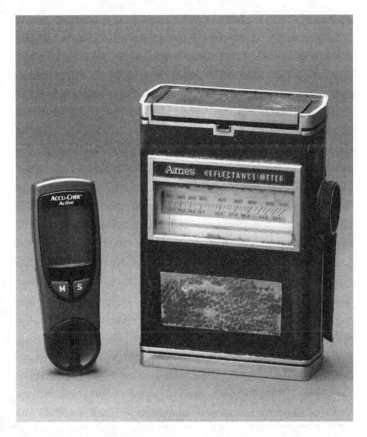

14. Ames Reflectance Meter (1970), the first device for measuring blood glucose outside the laboratory. On the left is one of the many meters available in 2000.

understand their disease and freed them from 'dirty' and uninformative urine tests. For anyone trying to keep blood sugars as near normal as possible, SMBG was essential, because, unlike urine tests, it gave warning of hypoglycaemia. It also gave them a target to aim for and enabled them to make informed therapeutic decisions. SMBG rapidly became popular, and improvements in technology mean that meters are now credit-card sized, require much less blood, and produce a result in ten seconds or less. Meters are cheap, whereas the strips remain expensive and are a major expense for the NHS: between 2001 and 2003 the cost of strips increased from £85 million to £118 million. Whether this is money well spent is controversial, since trials show that, especially in type 2 diabetes, SMBG does not improve glucose control compared to the much cheaper urine tests. Be this as it may, SMBG is popular with patients, and, as one of my colleagues commented: 'It may be possible to grope your way through a wood at night, but this is no reason for not using a flashlight if one is available!'[2]

The relationship of diabetes and HbA1c was discovered in 1968 by an Iranian doctor, Samuel Rahbar, who described what he thought was a new haemoglobin (the protein in red blood cells that carries oxygen). Rahbar analysed blood samples, which contained a variant that accounted for between 9 and 15 per cent of total haemoglobin. This was odd, because genetic variants (of which there are many) always constitute a fixed proportion. Rahbar found that people with this variant all had diabetes and later learned that it had been identified ten years earlier as HbA1c. In 1976 it was found that when diabetic patients had their blood-glucose levels kept normal in hospital, raised HbA1c concentrations returned to normal in four to six weeks. It was later shown that HbA1c was formed when glucose attached itself to haemoglobin and that the amount formed was proportional to the average blood glucose concentration over the 120-day life of the red cell. In other words, HbA1c could be used as a measure of the average blood glucose level over the previous six weeks.

The Diabetes Control and Complications Trial (DCCT)

The person who gave an enormous push to diabetes research in the USA was a TV producer, Lee Ducat, who founded the Juvenile Diabetes Foundation (JDF) in 1970 after her son developed diabetes. Frustrated by what she saw as the limited aims of the (doctor-dominated) ADA, she decided to raise money to find a cure. For her, lobbying congressmen was the way forward, since 'you could get more money for research in one day from the federal government than from years of fundraising'. As a result of her efforts, Congress instructed the director of the National Institutes of Health (NIH) to make a long-range plan for diabetes. One recommendation was a study of glucose control on the development of complications in type 1 diabetes. In 1985 the go-ahead was given for the DCCT, which compared the long-term effects of ordinary treatment (the control group) and near-normal blood sugars (the intensive-treatment group).

For the intensive-therapy group, several researchers had shown that, by using SMBG and either pumps or multiple injections of insulin, committed patients could achieve and maintain near-normal levels of blood glucose for months or years. More difficult was to decide how the control group should be treated. Ethically one could not simply reduce their insulin, and the worry was that enrolling people in a trial might improve their control so much that they would be indistinguishable from the intensive-treatment group—the so-called Hawthorne effect. If left to the care of their ordinary doctors, their blood sugars would probably be high, but the data were unlikely to be collected properly. The solution adopted was to find out the typical treatment of type 1 diabetes and mimic it. It turned out that in 1982 this meant seeing a doctor two or three times a year and being on one or two injections of short- and medium-acting insulin daily. Therefore, control patients in the DCCT were seen every three months by the investigators, who were not told the HbA1c value unless it was very high (over 13 per cent). No glucose targets were set, but the aim was freedom from symptoms and stable body weight.

In the intensively treated group, precise targets were set, and subjects measured blood glucose four or more times a day. For the whole trial they were seen at least once a month. The aim (achieved in only a few) was an HbA1c less than 6.05 per cent, the upper limit in people without diabetes. Between 1983 and 1989, 1,441 patients were recruited, and in 1993, after an average follow-up of 6.5 years, the study was stopped, because it was clear that intensive treatment was beneficial. It is a tribute to all involved that 99 per cent of patients completed the study.

A difference in average HbA1c was maintained throughout the study at 7.2 per cent in the intensively treated patients and 9.2 per cent in the conventional group. Intensive treatment reduced the risk of retinopathy by 76 per cent in those who did not have it at the beginning, and progression was reduced by 54 per cent in those who did. There were similar beneficial effects on kidney disease and neuropathy. Another important finding was that the benefit of intensive treatment increased over time. The 'cost' to the patient was three times more severe hypoglycaemia and an average weight gain of 4.6 kilograms, but importantly quality of life was not reduced. A smaller study in Sweden reached the same conclusions.

Thus, it was clear that intensive treatment was beneficial in type 1 diabetes, but it was by no means clear that the same would be true in the much commoner type 2, where obesity, hypertension, high cholesterol, and insulin resistance, singly or in combination, were as likely to influence the outcome as glucose control. The United Kingdom Prospective Diabetes Study provided a partial answer.

The United Kingdom Prospective Diabetes Study (UKPDS)

European diabetologists had never believed the results of the UGDP, but there was little will or money to repeat it. It is, therefore, extraordinary that, almost single-handedly, the Oxford physician Robert Turner (1938–99) started the UKPDS in 1977 and published the results in 1998. Finance was a constant problem, and the amount he originally asked for from the British Diabetic Association was, though small by American standards, half the charity's annual research budget. The trial involved 5,102 patients with newly diagnosed type 2 diabetes from 23 British hospitals. As in the DCCT, participants were divided into two groups. In the conventional (control) group the aim was a fasting blood glucose below 15 mmol/l (270 mg/dl) and in the intensive group a fasting level below 6 mmol/l (108 mg/dl). Two things became clear in the early years. The first was that after three months only 16 per cent of subjects reached the target fasting glucose of 6 mmol/l on diet alone, and only half of these maintained it for a year. The amount of weight loss necessary to control newly diagnosed type 2 diabetes was a surprise. Thus, those with an initial fasting plasma glucose of 6–8 mmol/l (108–144 mg/dl) had to lose 16 per cent of their pre-trial weight to reach the target of 6 mmol/l, while a 41 per cent loss was needed if the initial fasting glucose was 12–14 mmol/l (216–252 mg/dl). These findings would be confirmed later by the results of weight-loss surgery. A second finding, which had long been suspected by clinicians, was that over a period of five or more years type 2 diabetes got inexorably worse, in the sense that glucose levels rose and more drugs or larger doses had to be used to control them. Treatment with insulin and sulphonylureas was equally effective in keeping glucose levels down, although insulin was more likely to cause hypoglycaemia. To the surprise of many, metformin was equally good and did not cause weight gain or hypoglycaemia.

Over ten years, the average HbA1c was 7.9 per cent in the conventionally treated and 7.0 per cent in intensively treated patients. This small difference reduced the risk of any diabetes-related end points (microvascular, macrovascular, and cataract extraction) by 12 per cent and microvascular end points (predominantly retinal photocoagulation) by 25 per cent. There was no increase in cardiovascular deaths on sulphonylureas or insulin, which allayed previous fears that these agents were harmful. Unexpectedly, metformin in overweight patients reduced the risk of heart attacks. As in the DCCT, so in the UKPDS there turned out to be a legacy effect of good glucose control; a year after the end of the trial the difference of HbA1c between the groups was lost, but the benefits continued for ten years.

The UKPDS did not achieve particularly tight glucose control, and it seemed likely that lower would be better; for example, an HbA1c of 6 per cent would be better than 7 per cent. Therefore, in 2001 the NIH sponsored a trial (ACCORD) in 10,000 type 2 diabetics to compare ordinary treatment with an aggressive regimen to obtain HbA1c levels of 6 per cent or less. Unexpectedly, after an average of 3.5 years, the death rate was nearly a quarter higher in the intensive-treatment group. Confusingly, the rate of heart attacks was lower in the intensive group, but they were more likely to be fatal. The explanation of these results is not clear.

New drugs for type 2 diabetes

The UKPDS was planned in 1977 and used chlorpropamide and metformin, which by the 1990s were regarded as old-fashioned. However, the benefits of metformin in reducing cardiovascular deaths resulted in a renaissance for this drug, which had been available in Europe for more than thirty years but not licenced in the USA because of fears that, like phenformin, it might cause lactic acidosis. In 1994 it was marketed for the first time in America, where, protected by patent, it was thirty times more expensive than generic versions in Europe. The unique selling point of metformin was that it was the only drug that reduced insulin resistance until 1994, when troglitazone, the first of the thiazolidinediones (or glitazones), was launched. As the first new class of anti-diabetic drugs for forty years, these 'insulin sensitizers' caused great excitement in the diabetes community (stoked up by the drug companies). Their effect was hardly spectacular, with a reduction in HbA1c of 1 per cent or less in most trials, but market analysts expected them to become blockbusters. Within a year or two reports of serious liver damage began to appear, and troglitazone was withdrawn in England at the end of 1997. In 1999 it was followed onto the market by rosiglitazone and pioglitazone, which soon became best-sellers in spite of their side effects of weight gain, fluid retention, and heart failure. Rosiglitazone made about $3.2 billion a year until 2007, when a paper in the *New England Journal of Medicine* suggested that it increased the risk of heart attacks by 43 per cent. This caused a furore, and the shares of its maker dropped dramatically, as did sales of the drug. In 2008 the EASD and the ADA recommended that rosiglitazone not be used at all and relegated pioglitazone to a third-line treatment.

Traditionally doctors were reluctant to suggest insulin to people with type 2 diabetes, because it caused weight gain and also because most patients feared the needle and regarded injections as confirmation that their disease was reaching a terminal phase. When asked why she was so determined not to go onto insulin, a Bangladeshi woman said: 'Insulin means you have a very bad form of diabetes, which can lead to heart problems and kidney failure. I have heard that insulin is a last resort.' After the UKPDS, doctors and nurses made more effort to persuade their patients to start insulin earlier, and patients accepted injections more readily than had been anticipated.

It was probably this that persuaded one drug company, Amylin, that it was worth developing a new injectable anti-diabetic drug. It had been known for more than fifty years that glucose by mouth stimulated the pancreas to produce more insulin than an equivalent amount of glucose intravenously. This magnification was called the incretin effect and was assumed to be due to a hormone produced in the gut. Eventually the hormone was identified as glucagon-like peptide 1 (GLP-1), which not only stimulated insulin production but slowed stomach emptying and reduced appetite—exactly what the ideal anti-diabetic drug should do. Unfortunately it was broken down in the circulation within minutes by an enzyme called dipeptidyl dipeptidase (DDP IV). Amylin discovered that a venomous Arizona lizard, the Gila monster, had a form of GLP in its saliva. This was modified to make it last twelve hours and marketed as exanatide, which had to be injected twice daily but improved glucose control without weight gain. In 2008 the molecule was further modified to produce a once-weekly injection that reduced HbA1c by 1.9 per cent compared to 1.5 per cent with twice-daily injections. Another group of drugs (gliptins), which can be taken by mouth, were developed to block the activity of DPP IV, thereby increasing the concentration of natural GLP-1 in the blood.

Attacking atherosclerosis

The original aim of the UKPDS was to study blood-glucose control, but, when it was found that nearly half the patients had hypertension, a blood-pressure study was added in 1987. This compared tight blood-pressure control (144/82 mm Hg) with less tight (154/87 mm Hg). Tight control turned out to be very beneficial and reduced the risk of stroke by a third, diabetes-related death (heart attack or stroke) by a third, and deterioration of vision by a third. It is worth noting that nearly a third of patients who achieved the best blood-pressure control needed three anti-hypertensive drugs in addition to the two or more that were needed for blood-glucose control. To reduce cholesterol would require another pill, and from the late 1980s most diabetics were also advised to take aspirin, which reduces the stickiness of platelets and thereby cuts the risk of heart attacks.

Long before the UKPDS it was known that type 2 diabetics often had abnormal levels of fat, particularly cholesterol, in their blood. Many specialists doubted that reducing cholesterol would make much difference to the risk of heart disease, and their nihilism was bolstered by the fact that the drugs available were either ineffective or unpleasant to take. In the 1980s a new class of cholesterol-lowering drugs, the statins, were introduced, and the first trial in non-diabetic people with heart disease, the Scandinavian Simvastatin Survival Study (the 4S study) in 1994, showed that the relative risk of dying was reduced by 30 per cent in those taking simvastatin for five years. The benefit to diabetics with heart disease was greater, because of their greater absolute risk of having a heart attack. Makers of other statins were keen to get in on the action, and Pfizer funded a study (called CARDS) involving nearly 3,000 diabetics without heart disease. It was stopped in 2004 after only 3.9 years, because heart attacks had been reduced by 37 per cent and stroke by 48 per cent.

It was beginning to look as if attacking any component of the so-called metabolic syndrome—high glucose levels, high blood pressure, or high cholesterol—would reduce the frequency of heart disease and death, and it was natural to wonder whether tackling them simultaneously (multiple-risk-factor intervention) would be even better. There have been many such studies, but the most convincing is the Steno 2, started in Denmark in 1992. Patients enrolled had type 2 diabetes and microalbuminuria, the latter indicating damage to blood vessels and a high risk of heart attacks and other diabetic complications. During the thirteen years of follow-up, half the conventionally treated patients died, which underscores what a serious disease type 2 diabetes is once microalbuminuria has developed. Intensive treatment with blood-pressure- and cholesterol-lowering drugs reduced the risk of death by 20 per cent and the risk of developing nephropathy, retinopathy, and neuropathy by 50 per cent.

Treating microvascular complications

The DCCT (and clinical experience) showed that microvascular complications could be prevented by meticulous blood-glucose control, but in the real world few with either type 1 or type 2 achieved this and were not likely to. For example, in 2005–6 nearly a third of children and young people in the UK had an HbA1c over 9.5 per cent. An alternative strategy was to find how high glucose levels caused damage and then block the pathway. Two mechanisms have been investigated. The first involves an enzyme, aldose reductase, which converts glucose to sorbitol in nerves and the eye. In laboratory animals, drugs that blocked this enzyme (aldose reductase inhibitors) prevented nerve damage and cataracts. Unfortunately, in human diabetics they turned out to be ineffective and/or toxic.

A second putative mechanism was a process called glycosylation (or glycation), whereby glucose sticks to proteins (such as haemoglobin to form HbA1c). This occurs in tissues that do not need insulin to absorb glucose, such as the kidney, nerves, and blood vessels, and its magnitude is proportional to the amount of glucose in the blood. Glycosylation is also thought to be one mechanism of ageing, and it was hoped that blocking it would not only prevent diabetic complications but result in the holy grail of an anti-ageing drug. Vitamin E and aminoguanidine work in diabetic rats in the laboratory but only modestly or not at all in human beings. Neverthless both are advertised on the Internet as anti-ageing drugs.

One pharmacological success in treating complications was in impotence, which affected many diabetic men. The first effective treatment was in 1983, when a physiologist, Giles Brindley, showed that injecting the opiate papaverine into the penis caused an erection. This was memorable, not only because, unlike potions from sex shops, it worked, but also because of the way in which Brindley announced his discovery during a lecture to urologists in America. He had injected his penis fifteen minutes earlier, and, after showing a few slides, dropped his pants to reveal an impressive erection. Few diabetics were keen to inject their penis, and an alternative in the late 1980s was a vacuum pump that sucked blood into the penis. The erection was then maintained by a rubber band round the base of the penis. Apart from the palaver of interrupting lovemaking to use the machine, the main side effect was that the penis was cold.

The answer to some maidens' prayers, a pill to treat impotence (now called erectile dysfunction), came in 1998 from an unlikely source. A drug had been made a few years earlier at the Pfizer laboratories in Kent. It was originally tested as a treatment for angina and high blood pressure, but was found to have the (unexpected) side effect of producing erections. Pfizer therefore changed tack and developed it for the treatment of erectile dysfunction, for which it was approved in 1998 and marketed as Viagra. Where it scored over the alternative treatments was in terms of convenience, and, unlike them, the little blue pill was advertised for free in newspaper articles. In trials in diabetes it resulted in satisfactory erections in 50 per cent of men compared to only 10 per cent with dummy pills.

New insulins

After producing human insulin, the pharmaceutical industry set itself the goal of improving on nature by making faster-acting regular insulins and 'peakless' long-acting ones.

When injected subcutaneously, short-acting human insulins do not peak in the blood for thirty minutes, so that to reduce the glucose rise after a meal patients were advised to inject thirty minutes before eating. This was inconvenient, so few did. The reason for the delay is that, in solution, insulin molecules aggregate as hexamers (a six pack), and thirty minutes are needed for them to split into single molecules that can pass through the walls of blood vessels. By reversing the position of the last two amino acids of the B chain (proline and lysine), Eli Lilly scientists found that aggregation could be prevented. The resulting insulin lispro (1996) was absorbed faster, reached its peak faster, and was dissipated faster than ordinary human insulin. This meant that, if injected at the start of a meal, it reduced the glucose peak and also the risk of hypoglycaemia between meals. Novo had been in pole position in the race to produce a superfast insulin, until its Asp B10 was found to produce mammary tumours in rats, a salutary reminder that insulin is a growth factor and could potentially stimulate cell division and even cause cancer. By 1999 Novo had marketed its own fast-acting analogue, novorapid.

In tests on non-diabetic volunteers in the lab, lispro and novo-rapid did produce early peaks of insulin in the blood, and the difference from ordinary human insulin was obvious. Clinical trials in people with diabetes were less impressive, and most could not tell whether they were on ordinary insulin or the superfast variety. Nevertheless, and despite the fact that they were more expensive than 'ordinary' human insulin, fast-acting analogues were so successful that by 2006 they had 90 per cent of the market in Sweden, 87 per cent in the UK, and 75 per cent in France. In real-world conditions they did not produce much improvement in diabetic control in the generality of patients, in the same way that giving weekend golfers a set of expensive clubs does not make them world-beaters. There are many factors other than the type of insulin that affect the level of glucose control. At the time of writing (2009) there is some concern that the manufacturers may withdraw human insulin, leaving only analogues.

The first genetically engineered long-acting insulin was glargine, developed by Hoechst, and introduced in 2002. It precipitates in water at neutral pH, but is completely soluble in an acid solution. It is supplied as an acid solution (until the 1970s all insulins had been acid; neutral solutions were promoted as a great advance). After injection into the subcutaneous tissue, the solution is neutralized and the insulin precipitates, with small amounts being slowly released to produce a relatively constant blood level over twenty-four hours. On the back of intense marketing, glargine became a runaway financial success, although in practice its advantages over NPH, particularly for type 2 diabetics, were not great. In 2005 Novo Nordisk introduced another long-acting analogue, detemir. This has an attached fatty acid chain, which after injection binds to albumin in the blood. Both glargine and detemir show reduced day-to-day variability and reduced hypoglycaemia, particularly at night, compared to NPH.

Between 1980 and 2005 the insulin market expanded considerably because there were more people with diabetes, and more of those with type 2 were put on insulin to obtain the degree of control suggested by guidelines (for example, to maintain HbA1c below 7 per cent). As the market expanded, the number of manufacturers contracted, so that by 2000 the international market was controlled by three mega corporations: Eli Lilly, Novo Nordisk, and Sanofi-Aventis. It seems unlikely that any further modifications of the insulin molecule would improve subcutaneous insulin therapy, but what would be a massive hit would be an insulin that could be given in some way other than by injection. Possible routes could include the mouth, the nose, and the lungs.

Since 1980 many attempts have been made to protect insulin from being digested by enclosing it in various materials that it is hoped will pass intact through the stomach and then distintegrate in the small intestine. There have been many false dawns and headlines such as 'Insulin pill promises an end to the needle for diabetics' (*The Times*, 2007) make regular appearances.

Inhaled insulin did make it to the market in 2006 after eleven years in development, but was withdrawn after only a year. The makers Pfizer expected high demand and sales of $2 billion a year. Not only did there turn out to be far fewer needle phobics than anticipated, but the inhaler was cumbersome and dosage inflexible. In the event, it turned out that patients were not as keen as Pfizer had anticipated and payers were even less keen to pay £1,100 per year compared to £400 for injections.

IX

DIABETES BECOMES
EPIDEMIC

In the year 2000 the World Health Organization estimated that 171 million people worldwide had diabetes and
that by 2030 this would have increased to 366 million or
4.4 per cent of the total population. This chapter looks at how
we have arrived at this situation.

In Europe at the beginning of the twentieth century, diabetes at any age (but especially in the young) was uncommon in
hospitals. For example, at the Manchester Royal Infirmary from
1875 to 1895 there were only 272 cases among 27,721 medical
inpatients and in 1889–90 at the Berlin Charité hospital only 13
among 3,239. The main reason was that it was overwhelmingly
a disease of older, richer, and fatter people who were treated at
home; those who went to public hospitals were poor, under-
nourished, and relatively protected, because, as the English
physician Robert Saundby noted in 1897, 'diabetes is undoubtedly rare among people who lead a laborious life in the open
air, while it prevails chiefly with those who spend most of their
time in sedentary indoor occupations...there is no doubt that
diabetes must be regarded as one of the penalties of advanced
civilisation'.[1]

Much of the evidence that diabetes was a disease of the rich came from India. At a meeting on tropical diabetes in 1907, it was said that 'what gout is to the nobility of England, diabetes is to the aristocracy of India' and 'exercise, as a rule, is disliked by the gentlemen class of Bengal after a certain age'. The Indian experience suggested that mental work and excessive consumption of starches and sugars, aggravated by a completely sedentary life, were to blame. This was certainly true of the 'Bengali babu' (a clerk who could write English), 'whose girth had a great tendency to increase in direct proportion to any increment in his pay'. By contrast, diabetes was 'almost unknown among Hindu widows, who lead a most unexciting life, and are not indulged in excess of saccharine or other farinaceous foods'.[2]

Probably the first reference to an epidemic was in 1921, when Joslin talked about one in his hometown of Oxford, Massachusetts. Six of seven people in adjoining houses had died of diabetes, and he pointed out that, had they died of cholera, the public health authorities would have been round like a shot. As it was diabetes, nobody was particularly bothered. In the 1930s Joslin worked with the Metropolitan Life Insurance Company and established that the main risk factor for diabetes was being overweight. Environmental conditions were partly responsible, because, as Joslin wrote:

> The rapid expansion of the use of machines driven by mechanical power has made industrial workers mere tenders of machines, has lightened the burden of farm workers, transferred large numbers into clerical and sales jobs and reduced hours of labour. The amount of energy expended in work, therefore, has been drastically cut down for the majority of the working population. The growth of urban areas, often at the expense of the country, has made even larger numbers subject to these influences.[3]

The message about the consequences of an increasingly obese population was not only being preached by the puritanical and lean Dr Joslin. A writer in the *BMJ* in 1932 prophesied that, 'should the national overweight continue to grow unchecked, the mortality from the degenerative non-bacterial diseases will diminish the average expectation of life'.[4]

Look and you shall find

During the nineteenth century diabetes was defined as a condition in which there was sugar in the urine together with thirst, polyuria, and weight loss. It was not clear how to classify symptom-free people with sugar in their urine who were being discovered in increasing numbers during the first decades of the twentieth century as a result of tests for life insurance. Of more than 7,000 (male) applicants in New York between 1902 and 1907, 2.8 per cent had sugar in their urine, which meant automatic rejection by the insurance company but did not necessarily mean that they had diabetes. For a definitive diagnosis it was necessary to measure blood glucose. This was expensive and required much skill and time and large volumes of blood until 1912, when Ivar Christian Bang (1869–1918) invented a method that needed only a fingerprick. This made it possible to do multiple measurements over a few hours, and was used to investigate the effects of various foods or glucose drinks on the blood sugar of normal people and diabetics. In 1913 a Danish physician, Åge Th. B. Jacobsen (1885–1979), was one of the first to describe the effect of drinking 100 grams of glucose in water (later called a glucose-tolerance test or GTT); normal people's blood sugar rose within 5 minutes, peaked at about 30, and returned to baseline in 100 minutes.

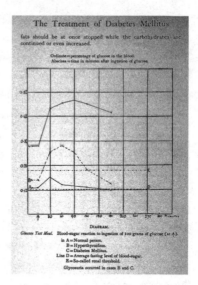

The Treatment of Diabetes Mellitus

fats should be at once stopped while the carbohydrates are continued or even increased.

Ordinate = percentage of glucose in the blood.
Abscissa = time in minutes after ingestion of glucose.

DIAGRAM.

Glucose Test Meal. Blood-sugar reaction to ingestion of 100 grams of glucose (at ↑).
in A = Normal person.
B = Hyperthyroidism.
C = Diabetes Mellitus.
Line D = Average fasting level of blood-sugar.
E = So-called renal threshold.
Glycosuria occurred in cases B and C.

15. Stylised glucose tolerance test results from the *Edinburgh Medical Journal* 1921. (*Wellcome Library, London*)

Jacobsen found that four of six pregnant women had glucose in their urine, in spite of a normal or subnormal blood glucose. This harmless glycosuria of pregnancy is now known to be common and is due to a lowering of the renal threshold whereby glucose spills into the urine when blood levels are normal. Clinicians also knew of apparently healthy people who always had glucose in their urine. In 1917 George Graham in London reported five cases including a 28-year-old army captain who first tested his urine in 1908 at the age of 20 and found sugar. He did the test because a year earlier both his brother and sister had been found to have glycosuria. The 23-year-old sister was strictly dieted for three years, but felt ill and lost weight. She therefore returned to normal eating and remained well, even during pregnancy. This relatively uncommon condition, which

Graham called *diabetes innocens*, is now called renal glycosuria and is usually inherited.

Increasing use of the GTT showed that some older people without diabetic symptoms had strikingly high blood sugars after drinking glucose and after meals. One doctor in 1921 described them as living 'in a state of persistent hyperglycaemia', although, as he pointed out, this could be corrected by simple dietary and lifestyle advice. This state (a relatively normal fasting blood sugar with high sugars after meals) was often called 'alimentary glycosuria' and was distinguished from diabetes because of the absence of symptoms. It emphasized the difficulty of interpreting the GTT and distinguishing diabetes from normality. In the 1920s it was agreed that the normal fasting glucose level was under 120 mg/dl (6.7 mmol/l) and that, in health, blood sugar returned to the fasting level within two hours after drinking glucose. How high the intermediate values could be without indicating diabetes was much disputed. As late as 1975 an epidemiologist Kelly West (1925–80) asked twenty prominent diabetes specialists (eleven American) what two-hour level in the glucose tolerance test they would consider abnormal. All quoted a wide range for the lowest values that they considered 'clearly abnormal' (130–200 mg/dl or 7.2–11.1 mmol/l) and the highest that were 'clearly normal' (110–180 mg/dl or 6.1–10.0 mmol/l). These differences of opinion arose because population surveys (discussed later in the chapter) showed that, in the general public, blood glucose was distributed as a continuous variable, with no clear dividing line between normal and abnormal (as is also the case with blood pressure and serum cholesterol). Something that was often ignored was the lack of reproducibility of the GTT, which was discovered in 1927 by a New York doctor, William Lennox. He found that a quarter of 140 people with epilepsy had a 'pre-diabetic' curve. Unable to explain this, he repeated the tests and found that half had now become normal. Lennox did further repeat tests on medical students and people with epilepsy and found that a second GTT was almost always lower than the first. Many others subsequently confirmed his findings. Another confounding factor was the previous diet. It is not clear who first showed that starvation lowers the tolerance of man or animals to glucose, but it was well known in the nineteenth century that it caused what was called 'vagabond diabetes', and in 1913 Bang showed that starvation for a few days caused high blood sugars in the GTT. This was repeatedly rediscovered over the next fifty years, with the warning that people who were to have a GTT should eat 300 grams of carbohydrate a day for the previous three days.

The GTT showed that people could have diabetes without having symptoms, and from a public health standpoint it was important to find out how large the submerged part of the iceberg was. After the Second World War it seemed that diabetes was becoming more common, and between 1947 and 1962 attempts were made to screen total communities. The motivation behind these studies varied. Some were part of public-health initiatives, while others were research projects by diabetes specialists. The assumption was that early detection would lead to prompt and effective treatment and stop the disease getting worse. The first diabetes-detection drive was in 1947 in Joslin's birthplace, Oxford, Massachusetts, where two-thirds of the population of this small town were tested. Previously diagnosed diabetes was found in 40 people, previously undiagnosed diabetes in 30, and blood sugars in 25 were abnormal but not high enough to be labelled diabetic. The total prevalence of diabetes was 1.7 per cent. A follow-up study in 1950 confirmed these findings and added the information that people with 'a little sugar in the urine' or blood-sugar levels 'a little higher than normal' developed diabetes eight times more often than those with normal blood sugars. In the 1953 follow-up, participants had a full medical examination, which showed that abnormalities of the eyes, heart, and blood vessels in the leg were much commoner in people with diabetes. Surveys were also done in Bergen, Norway (1957), Ibstock, England (1957), and Birmingham, England (1963) with similar results. All found people with blood sugars that were not normal but were not sufficiently high to meet the accepted definition of diabetes. They were called latent or borderline diabetics until 1979, when their condition was renamed impaired glucose tolerance or IGT.

One of the most important studies in teasing out the causes of coronary artery disease in general and in diabetes in particular was started in 1950 in Framingham, a town of 28,000 people near Boston, Massachusetts. After those who already had heart disease had been weeded out, the aim was to follow more than 5,000 healthy men and women aged 30 to 60 for twenty years. Diabetes affected 1.92 per cent of the population and, in sixteen years of follow-up, their mortality from heart disease was three times that of the general population. The relative excess among diabetic women (confined to those on insulin) was particularly striking. Diabetics also had significantly more non-fatal heart attacks and were more likely to suffer from angina. The annual rate of new intermittent claudication (pain in the calves on walking, which is due to narrowing of the arteries) in diabetics was five times higher in men and eight times higher in women, compared to the general population. In 1961 the leader of the study Thomas Dawber (1913–2005) put forward the concept of risk factors for heart disease and identified the major ones as high blood pressure, high cholesterol levels, irregularities in heart rhythm, and diabetes. This led to an important change in medical practice. Traditionally people went to the doctor because they had symptoms—for example, headache, breathlessness, and blurred vision. With this group of symptoms, examination might show a blood pressure of 220/150 mm Hg and the diagnosis would be malignant hypertension. As a result of the Framingham findings, risk factors for cardiovascular disease were used to redefine hypertension and diabetes from diseases with symptoms and pathological signs to diseases that could be detected only by laboratory tests—what I call 'diseases the doctor says you have got' as opposed to 'diseases you know you've got' and what the press call 'silent killers'.[5] An important part of the management of diabetes today is screening for risk factors for heart disease and treating them. Healthy levels of all the risk factors have progressively been revised downwards. In the late 1990s the definition of diabetes was changed from a fasting blood glucose of over 7.8 mmol/l to over 7.0 (140–126 mg/dl), thus greatly increasing the number of patients.

The Framingham and other studies in Western populations documented gradually increasing levels of diabetes between 1950 and 1970, albeit from a low baseline of around 1 per cent. Rapidly modernizing populations elsewhere had explosive increases. The first indication of the effect of 'Westernization' was in the Pima Indians of Arizona. In the eighteenth and nineteenth centuries these Native Americans irrigated the desert to create productive farms. In the early twentieth century European settlers diverted the water, and the Pimas' agriculture collapsed, so that they were forced from a subsistence economy and became dependent on welfare benefits. Their traditional high-fibre diet of beans and vegetables was replaced by a high-fat, highly refined diet. Having no work, they indulged liber-ally in alcohol and spent time lounging about and driving old cars. Diabetes was rare in the 1930s and in the early 1950s only 3 per cent of the population were affected. Thereafter obesity and diabetes increased inexorably, so that by 1990 the Pimas had become very fat, with diabetes affecting 37 per cent of men and 54 per cent of women. Today the disease dominates their lives, and they await fatalistically for the almost inevitable kid-ney failure, heart attacks, and amputations. There is a group of Pimas in Northern Mexico, thought to have split from those in Arizona around 1,000 years ago, who pursue a traditional life-style and are thin. Their diet, like that of the Arizona Pimas 100 years ago, consists mainly of beans, corn, and potatoes, grown by traditional techniques involving hard work. A small survey in 1994 found that diabetes was nearly eight times less common in Mexican Pimas than among their distant relatives in Arizona.

The inhabitants of Nauru, a small, isolated, coral island in the South Pacific (population 9,265 in 2006), vie with the Pimas for the dubious distinction of the world's highest rate of diabetes. Nauru has (or had) large deposits of phosphate, which became the only export and made the islanders so rich that by the 1960s their per capita income was one of the highest in the world. As a result, they abandoned agriculture and lived on imported (usu-ally energy-dense) food. They also gave up walking and used motorbikes or cars to move around the 20-square-kilometre island. By 1976 a third of all adults had diabetes, a disease that had been almost unknown twenty years earlier. As with the Pimas, obesity went hand in hand with diabetes. Unfortunately, being fat was seen, as is still the case in many countries, as a sign of success, and Nauru even had a Big is Beautiful Pageant! By the beginning of the twenty-first century the phosphate deposits

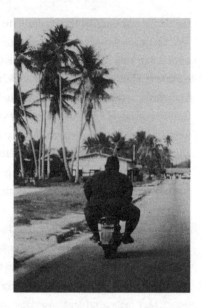

16. Fat Nauruan on a motor bike. (*Courtesy of Professor Paul Zimmet*).

had been exhausted, much of the money generated by them had been squandered by the government, and 45 per cent of the population, including even teenagers, had type 2 diabetes. With this came heart disease and kidney failure, so that life expectancy is only 58 years for men and 65 for women.

The plague of diabetes struck the Pimas and Nauruans (as well as native Australians and the people of Papua New Guinea) even while they stayed put, but in other populations the driving force was migration, either internally from the countryside to the city or into another country. Migrants from the Indian subcontinent have a remarkable susceptibility to diabetes, whether they move to Fiji, Mauritius, Singapore, the USA, or Britain, and in all these places they have more diabetes than the indigenous population. The prevalence of diabetes in rural India is about 2 per cent and rises to 8 per cent in the cities. Those who have emigrated to a 'Westernized' environment have rates four or five times higher, which are reached within only two decades in the new environment. The story of Chinese who emigrate to Hong Kong, Mauritius, and Singapore is similar. These are worrying observations because of the large number of people in India and China who will develop diabetes as they exercise less and eat more, especially processed food, in their rapidly modernizing homelands. In 1994, 7 million Chinese had diabetes, by 2003 this had risen to 30 million, and is expected to rise above 45 million by 2020.

It is not only Pima Indians or South Pacific islanders who become fat when food is plentiful. Evolution has not fitted humans with a mechanism for disposing of excess energy (or calories), because there was no need for one during the millennia when food was scarce. The priority in evolutionary terms was to lay down fat in times of plenty as an insurance against famine. The weight of US citizens (and to a lesser extent those of other developed countries) increased progressively over the last two decades of the twentieth century, so that by 2003 17 per cent of adolescents and 32 per cent of adults in the USA were obese. The reasons are easy to identify but difficult to deal with. Children and adults take less exercise, spend a lot of time watching television or playing computer games, are assaulted by advertisements for 'unhealthy' foods, and eat larger portions. This epidemic of obesity has spawned a new disease—type 2 diabetes in children and adolescents, which should not be confused with MODY (see Prologue). The worry, and expectation, is that these 'children' will develop severe complications in twenty years—that is, in their 30s or early 40s. The prevalence of this new disease is increasing rapidly in the USA and Europe, and among black and Hispanic adolescents in the USA it is probably more common than type 1 diabetes.

It would be wrong to give the impression that type 2 diabetes is simply the result of obesity and a sedentary lifestyle, important though these are. Inheritance is also important.

Heredity

The ancient Hindus knew that diabetes often ran in families, and diabetes specialists in the nineteenth century noted that about a quarter of their patients had other affected family members. The field of human genetics was founded in the early 1900s with the rediscovery of the work of the Moravian monk Gregor Mendel (1822–84), but the only examples of Mendelian inheritance in man were rare conditions such as short fingers (dominant), colour blindness (X-linked recessive), and alkaptonuria (recessive). These conditions all result from single gene mutations. Commoner diseases such as diabetes and hypertension that clearly had an inherited component did not follow Mendelian rules, because, as we now realize, they are not due to single genes. Early work on the inheritance of diabetes consisted in reports of unusual families with (unsuccessful) attempts to fit them into recessive, dominant, or X-linked recessive patterns. It was an important advance when in 1933 Gregory Pincus and Priscilla White in Boston devised methods for pooling family histories and testing the findings against various Mendelian hypotheses. On the basis of the family histories of 523 patients and 153 non-diabetic controls, they suggested that the data were most consistent with simple autosomal recessive inheritance, whereby each unaffected parent (a heterozygote or carrier) contributes one copy of the abnormal gene so that the child (a homozygote) has a full complement of abnormal genes, which cause the disease. The commonest autosomal recessive disease in the early twenty-first century is cystic fibrosis. Joslin assumed recessive inheritance for the genetic counselling that he offered his patients. A flavour of his paternalistic approach is shown by a paper in 1935, where he began with the following case history:

> An attractive young woman comes to your office and asks you if she can get married. A moment's conversation suffices to disclose that she is unusually intelligent; she is evidently physically strong, because she is a champion tennis player, often rides to hounds for six hours at a time, has driven an automobile recently 300 miles in a day, and repeatedly dances all night. In the midst of city gaieties she has learned stenography and typewriting and, what is more, secured a job.

This 21-year-old superwoman has had diabetes for fourteen years and 'has never been so careless as to develop [ketoacidotic] coma'. Joslin did what he thought any father would and asked: (1) Is he a good boy? (2) Is he really in love, and are you too? (3) Can I examine him physically and mentally and decide whether he is good enough for you, because I have known you for fourteen years? (4) Are you sure neither he nor his relatives have diabetes? (5) Do his parents know you have diabetes? (6) Do your parents approve? (7) Are there funds enough to take care of you, if you are ill, and to provide exceptional attention in a hospital if you should ever become pregnant? (8) Does this young man realize that he must take unusual care of you and help you to keep your diabetes controlled? Presumably some young men actually underwent this grilling! If they did and the answers were satisfactory, Joslin would have said 'get married and God bless you'. He added a further statement about the superpeople with diabetes:

[I] must say that I do admire the backbone and the brains of the average diabetic and I truly believe on the whole they are superior to the common run of people and therefore their good qualities merit cultivation. Second, I think they are less apt to drink, far less likely to have syphilis or gonorrhea, and distinctly less likely to have, what is anathema to me, 'nervous prostration and nerves'.[6]

Further studies over the next thirty years only led to increasing confusion, with virtually every possible mode of inheritance being suggested. All were based on the postulate that there was a single gene that determined whether someone got diabetes or not, and it was usually assumed that diabetes in the young and old was a single disease. The geneticist Harry Harris (1919–94) studied the family histories of a large group of patients at King's College Hospital in 1947 and 1948 and came up with the intuitively attractive theory that juvenile diabetes was caused by homozygosity (inheritance of two copies of the abnormal gene) and the adult-onset form by heterozygosity (one copy). The difficulties of collecting large numbers of comprehensive family histories prevented the collection of new data, so that many were reanalysed using increasingly elaborate statistical techniques; this often showed that the original data could also support opposite conclusions. For example, the data of Harris cited above was thought by Arthur Steinberg (1912–2006) to be compatible with autosomal recessive inheritance. One corollary of the autosomal recessive theory was that anyone with two diabetic parents was certain to develop diabetes, and in 1965 the World Health Organization advised that two people with diabetes should not marry one another or, if they did marry, should not have children. Critics of this gratuitous piece of advice pointed out that whether diabetics married other diabetics or non-diabetics would make very little difference to the total number in the population—if only because, if diabetics marry each other, the number available to marry non-diabetics is halved.

In 1965 another geneticist, Jim Neel (1915–2000) of the University of Michigan, crystallized the sense of frustration by referring to diabetes as the geneticist's nightmare and asking rhetorically: 'Why after this dreary recital would any geneticist even venture into this obviously genetically unprofitable area? The answer is very simple. This is a relatively common and potentially fatal disorder in which there is much evidence for a family predisposition.'[7]

The main tenet of Darwinism is that genes that give their possessors an advantage in the struggle for survival are the ones that persist. It was, therefore, a paradox that a genetic disease such as diabetes with no discernible biological advantage should be so common. Neel put forward a hypothesis of what he called a 'thrifty genotype rendered detrimental by progress'. He suggested that the basic defect was 'a quick insulin trigger', which in hunter-gatherers with their feast–famine lifestyle would mean that food could be stored in times of plenty. Whether Neel's theory is right (probably not in the detail), the genetic make-up of our palaeolithic ancestors was selected during 30,000 years in relation to a diet that was very different from that of modern man. A third of hunter-gatherers' food is protein with a very low fat content, because game animals are lean, as must have been their muscular and fit human predators. Their carbohydrate intake would have varied, but certainly contained a lot of fibre. They would also, in common with all other mammals, have ingested more potassium than sodium. This is relevant, because a high salt or sodium intake is one factor leading to high blood pressure.

Current humans still have the palaeolithic genotype, and, in those who continue with the traditional lifestyle, diabetes, high blood pressure, and atherosclerosis are vanishingly rare. However, as we have seen with the Pimas and Nauruans, when a traditional society, whether by migration or acculturation, adopts a Western lifestyle, with a salt-rich, high-energy diet and lack of exercise, everything changes.

I have suggested that the genetic constitution that predisposes to diabetes is one that has been selected over many thousands of years for its ability to withstand intermittent starvation. In the case of South Pacific islanders, this occurred on long inter-island voyages, which only those with the 'diabetes-prone' genetic constitution survived. When exposed to abundant food, this constitution leads not only to overweight and diabetes but also to high blood pressure and abnormal levels of fat in the blood. In 1988 in a lecture to the American Diabetes Association, Gerald Reaven (b. 1928) drew attention to the simultaneous occurrence of these 'diseases of civilization'.[8] He originally called this syndrome X, although it is now more usually called the metabolic syndrome. Reaven suggested that the underlying abnormality was insulin resistance, the commonest cause of which is obesity. In most societies the increase in diabetes (and associated components of the metabolic syndrome) in the last decade of the twentieth century and the first decade of the twenty-first has been paralleled by a rise in obesity. It is not body fat *per se* but its distribution that determines diabetes and the metabolic syndrome. In 1947 a French physician Jean Vague distinguished between gynaecoid (female) and android (male) obesity. The former, where fat is deposited on the hips and buttocks, is harmless. Male pattern obesity (the beer belly) can also occur in women and is bad. What is particularly important is

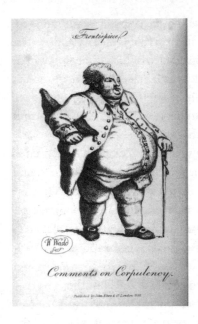

17. 1829 drawing of a man with abdominal obesity. Until the easy availability of processed foods towards the end of the 20th century, this type of obesity signified wealth and still does in some countries. (*Wellcome Library, London*)

the amount of intra-abdominal fat, which can be estimated by measuring the waist–hip ratio and measured directly with an MRI scanner.

How will we stop the diabetes epidemic?

It will now be clear that type 2 diabetes results when a particular genetic constitution is exposed to obesity and lack of exercise. We cannot change people's genes, but lifestyle modification in those at risk is possible and has been successful in small groups. In an American study, the Diabetes Prevention Program (DPP) over 3,000 middle-aged people (two-thirds women) with obesity and impaired glucose tolerance were treated with a weight losing diet and either placebo or metformin or 150 minutes of exercise per week. During nearly three years of follow-up, diet and exercise reduced the incidence of diabetes by 58 per cent and metformin reduced it by 31 per cent. Smaller studies in China (1997) and Finland (2001) reached similar conclusions.

Genetic factors play a part in obesity, but pictures of starving populations make it clear that everyone will lose weight if they take in fewer calories than they burn. The problem is that in a free society with abundant food willpower is also necessary, and this is where individuals are usually found wanting, even with the help of physicians and dieticians. Those who complete hospital weight-loss programmes (less than half of those who enrol) lose only 10 per cent of body weight and most regain it within one or two years.

One proven way of losing weight is with surgery. Operations can either reduce the capacity of the stomach (gastric banding) or bypass part of the intestine so that food is not absorbed properly (Roux-en-Y gastric bypass). Both cause permanent weight loss of 50–75 per cent, which cures type 2 diabetes in three-quarters of patients and impaired glucose tolerance in all. Unfortunately, operations are expensive and potentially hazardous. A pill that would do the same is much more attractive, and every year Americans spend $45 billion on non-prescription weight-loss products. Not surprisingly, the pharmaceutical industry is keen to find an effective and safe weight-reducing drug, which would be a huge money spinner, especially if it had to be taken indefinitely to keep the weight off. Fifty years of searching for this particular cash cow have been a major disappointment. Most drugs used up to 1990 were derivatives of amphetamine. Their record was not good; some were addictive, and others had serious side effects, such as heart-valve damage and pulmonary hypertension. Three new drugs were developed in the 1990s: orlistat prevents the absorption of fat but has the side effect of oily faeces and faecal incontinence, sibutramine is an appetite suppressant, and rimombinant blocks cannabinoid receptors in the brain through which marijuana and chemicals produced in the body stimulate appetite. These drugs are only marginally effective. A 2007 review of thirty studies in which orlistat, sibutramine, and rimombinant were taken for a year found an average weight loss of less than 5 kilograms, with 30–40 per cent of those taking them dropping out before the end of the study.

From a public-health point of view the question is whether we should be trying to find drugs to 'cure' obesity or whether we should devote our efforts to changing the 'obesogenic' environment. It is difficult to see how we could do the latter in a free society. One can exhort people to walk more but cannot force them. We can wring our hands about the power of advertisers of high-energy snacks but cannot ban them, and the same goes for increasing portion sizes—between 1970 and the 1990s a typical snack increased from 160 to 250 calories and a soft drink from 130 to 200.

POSTSCRIPT

There is a tendency to think of progress in diabetes in terms of new drugs, new insulins, and other technological developments on which I have concentrated, perhaps excessively. Patients need effective tools, but there is much more to managing diabetes than having the newest glucose meter or newest insulin. The support of one's family and a medical team is also critical, as Allen (of under-nutrition fame) recognized when he wrote in 1962: 'The requisites for the diabetic therapist are time and detailed attention. No doctor can control a host of patients on an assembly-line basis. While a nurse or dietician may help, the doctor must have close acquaintance with his patient and give ample time to his problems, or refer him to somebody else who will do so.'[1] Until the 1970s, care in England was almost exclusively provided in hospital clinics staffed by doctors, with the token presence of a dietician and possibly a social worker. These clinics ran like production lines, where the doctor sat in judgement and dispensed advice about what or, more usually, what not to do.

Patients' views were not solicited, and the idea that they might have any input in designing their regimen was unthinkable. The doctor in charge expected his instructions to be followed to the letter and blamed the patient when the desired level of glucose control was not obtained. This was unsurprising, because he (and it was usually he) had been trained to diagnose and treat acute illnesses such as pneumonia and heart attacks, where

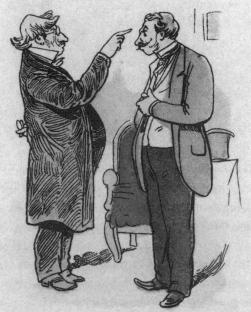

— Plus de farineux, plus de sucre, et
ne pas boire... surtout ne pas boire...
tout est là.
   Après tout, il y a tant de gens qui ne
         meurent pas du diabète...
               comme Cornélius....

18. Doctor lecturing a patient about what not to eat. "No more bread, no more sugar, don't drink...above all don't drink...after all many people don't die of diabetes." (*Wellcome Library, London*)

patient input was irrelevant. Those with the most experience in managing chronic disease were GPs, who had been deskilled by the expectation that diabetes would be managed in a hospital clinic. During the late 1970s it gradually came to be accepted that a more holistic model of care might work better than the authoritarian one. In 1982 the chest physician Charles Fletcher, who by then had had diabetes for forty years, wrote:

> We doctors who have to manage chronic disabling conditions should pay far more attention to the importance to patients of their being independent of as many restrictions as possible, and we should encourage them to be original in their self management. We should more often ask the question 'How do you feel about your illness?' or 'What bothers you most about your treatment?'[2]

When chided about their failure to do this, most doctors would probably have pointed out that their clinic was already overloaded and that asking people about their emotional life risked opening Pandora's box. Nevertheless, things were changing. In 1979 a group of younger doctors, including Jean-Phillipe Assal of Geneva and Michael Berger (1944–2002) of Dusseldorf, both of whom had studied at the Joslin Clinic in Boston, set up a European Diabetes Education Study Group (DESG) to explore new methods of patient education. During the 1980s, in his home base of Dusseldorf and in several (at that time communist) East European countries, Berger tested a system in which people with type 1 diabetes ate normal meals and were taught to match insulin doses to the amount of food while keeping their blood glucose close to normal. To the surprise of many, this produced sustained improvements in blood-glucose control without increasing severe hypoglycaemia. Despite its success, Berger's system was ignored elsewhere until introduced to England in 2002 under the acronym DAFNE (Dose Adjustment For Normal Eating). Most people who have taken part in DAFNE courses are delighted with their new-found freedom, but history tells us that there is never anything really new. In 1986 Jack Eastwood, a retired headmaster, wrote an article in the

BMJ remembering that when he developed diabetes in 1925 at the age of 13 he was

> taken to a Harley Street specialist and spent three weeks in a nursing home, during which time my diet and insulin requirements were settled. I returned home to be looked after by my parents in accordance with the detailed instructions given to them. My diet was strictly controlled, especially on the carbohydrate side: for two years all my food was weighed and no excesses at all were allowed.[3]

In 1931 he won a scholarship to New College, Oxford, and once there decided to use a less orthodox method of treatment. He ate lunch in an ordinary restaurant, played golf nearly every afternoon (such was university life in the 1930s!), and then had a normal four-course dinner in hall. Before each meal he injected 'the amount of insulin that I knew from experience would be needed to cope with the food about to be eaten, due allowance being made for what I expected to be doing during the next few hours'. In 1935 he visited a specialist for the last time and was told there was no need to go again, since he knew more about controlling his own diabetes than the specialist. Once or twice he wondered whether to switch from multiple injections of soluble insulin to something 'more modern', but decided there was no point in changing a system that worked so well. I did not know Jack Eastwood, but I had many extraordinarily resourceful patients like him from whom I learned as much as I did from my formal teachers.

GLOSSARY

ACE INHIBITOR shorthand for angiotensin-converting enzyme Inhibitor, a type of blood-pressure-lowering drug; their chemical names end in –pril-e.g. captopril

ADDISON'S DISEASE adrenal cortical failure most commonly caused by autoimmunity

AMINO ACID a group of chemical compounds that are critical to life; twenty different amino acids form the building blocks of proteins

ANGIOGRAPHY injection of opaque material into blood vessels so that they can be seen on an x-ray

ANTIGEN a substance that stimulates the formation of an antibody

AUTOIMMUNE DISEASE a condition in which antibodies are formed to a normal constituent of the body—e.g. the thyroid gland or islets of Langerhans

ALBUMINURIA albumin (a protein) in the urine; the same as proteinuria

ATHEROSCLEROSIS or **ATHEROMA** hardening of the arteries

AUTOSOMAL RECESSIVE a type of inheritance in which the disease develops only if the child receives a copy of the abnormal gene from both parents; the best-known example is cystic fibrosis

BRITTLE DIABETES a term used to denote type 1 diabetes, which is so difficult to control that the patient is repeatedly admitted to hospital with ketoacidosis

BIGUANIDES a class of anti-diabetic drugs that reduces insulin resistance; the only one still in use is metformin

C-PEPTIDE the chain of amino acids that connects the two chains of insulin during its manufacture in the beta cells

CALORIE a measure of energy: 1 gram of carbohydrate gives 4 calories, 1 gram of protein 4, and 1 gram of fat 9

CAPSAICIN CREAM a counter-irritant produced from chilli peppers; used for acute painful neuropathy

CATARACT loss of transparency of the cornea of the eye; diabetes is a common cause

CUSHING'S SYNDROME overactivity of the cortex of the adrenal gland, most commonly as a result of a pituitary tumour; a moon face and diabetes are two of the clinical features

DIABETES INSIPIDUS a disease caused by lack of anti-diuretic hormone; the main symptom is excessive urination

DIPEPTIDYL DIPEPTIDASE (DDP IV) an enzyme that destroys GLP 1 in the circulation; gliptins are drugs developed to block this enzyme

DROPSY an old name for generalized oedema or swelling

ENDOCRINE GLAND a gland that discharges its product into the bloodstream; examples are the thyroid and adrenal glands, as well as the islets of Langerhans

EXOCRINE GLAND a gland that discharges its product via a duct into a body cavity; examples are the salivary glands, the lachrmyal (tear-producing) glands, and most of the pancreas.

FASTING BLOOD SUGAR or GLUCOSE the level of blood sugar on waking after no food has been eaten overnight

FIBRE or DIETARY FIBRE sometimes called roughage; the indigestible part of vegetables that prevents constipation

GANGRENE death of tissue, usually as a result of inadequate blood supply

GASTROPARESIS paralysis of emptying of the stomach as a result of nerve damage

GESTATIONAL DIABETES abnormally high blood glucose levels during pregnancy; usually comes on after the sixth month and goes away after delivery; usually has no symptoms

GLITAZONES a class of anti-diabetic drugs that reduce insulin resistance; examples are pioglitazone and rosiglitazone

GLUCOSE also sometimes called grape sugar; the main source of energy for the cells of the body

GLUCOSE TOLERANCE TEST a test for diagnosing diabetes, in which 75 grams of glucose in solution are drunk, and blood glucose concentrations measured for 2, 3, or 5 hours; the test was once used extensively, but is nearly obsolete in the twenty-first century

GLUCAGON a hormone that raises blood glucose, produced by the alpha cells of the islets of Langerhans

GLYCOGEN a compound (polymer) made in the liver or muscles from thousands of glucose molecules; the primary form of short-term energy storage

GLYCOSURIA glucose in the urine

HAEMOGLOBIN AIC a glycosylated form of haemoglobin that can be used as a measure of blood-glucose control

HYPERGLYCAEMIA a higher than normal level of glucose in the blood; a normal fasting level is below 7 mmol/l and a normal random level below 11

HYPERTENSION high blood pressure

HYPOGLYCAEMIA a lower than normal level of blood glucose—i.e. below 3.5mmol/l

HYPOPHYSECTOMY removal of the pituitary gland

INTERNAL SECRETION the old name for hormones

IMMUNOSUPPRESSION a reduction of the potency of the immune system, which is artificially induced by drugs to prevent rejection of an organ transplant; a side effect is to reduce the defence against infection, which also depends on the immune system

IMMUNOASSAY a method of measuring small quantities of biological substances such as hormones by using antibodies against them

INTERCAPILLARY GLOMERULOSCLEROSIS the specific kidney disease in diabetes

ISLET CELL ANTIBODY an autoantibody against the beta cells of the islets of Langerhans

KETOACIDOSIS acidification of the blood caused by the breakdown of fats to ketones as a result of insulin deficiency

LIPOATROPHY dissolving of fat at the site of insulin injections to leave unsightly hollows

LIPOHYPERTROPHY fatty lumps at the site of insulin injections

MACROSOMIA literally large body—a term used for a baby weighing over 4,000 grams

MACULAR OEDEMA the macula is the part of the retina responsible for sharp vision; oedema or swelling is caused by leakage from blood vessels damaged by diabetes

MATURITY ONSET DIABETES old name for type 2 diabetes

METABOLIC SYNDROME a combination of abnormalities, including diabetes, hypertension, hyperlipidaemia, and obesity, which originate from insulin resistance and cause heart disease

METABOLISM the biochemical processes that maintain life; one form of metabolism involves changing food into energy

MICROVASCULAR COMPLICATIONS the diabetic complications that are the result of damage to small blood vessels— retinopathy, nephropathy, and neuropathy

MICROALBUMINURIA a low concentration of albumin (protein) in the urine—the earliest sign of kidney damage

MODY acronym for Maturity Onset type Diabetes of the Young, an inherited form of diabetes in the young that is distinct from type 1; it is dominantly inherited, so that half the children of a sufferer will also have it

MUTATION a change in a gene

MYXOEDEMA old term for hypothyroidism; like other autoimmune endocrine diseases, more common with type 1 diabetes

NEPHROPATHY disease of the kidney; in the first half of the twentieth century, the term 'nephritis' was used

OPHTHALMOSCOPE an instrument for examining the retina at the back of the eye

ORGANOTHERAPY or **OPOTHERAPY** an old term for the use of animal extracts to treat disease; we would now talk about endocrine replacement therapy

PERIPHERAL NEURITIS an old name for peripheral neuropathy—damage to nerves outside the brain and spinal cord

PHOTOCOAGULATION the use of light to make burns on the retina as a treatment for retinopathy; in the twenty-first century these burns are made with a laser, and we talk about laser treatment

PROGESTERONE a female sex hormone produced in the ovaries

PHTHISIS old name for tuberculosis

POLYDIPSIA excessive thirst

POLYURIA excessive urination

POLYPHAGIA excessive appetite

PROINSULIN the precursor to insulin in the beta cells; it consists of insulin and C peptide

PROLIFERATIVE RETINOPATHY the most severe form of diabetic retinopathy in which new blood vessels grow on the retina and bleed into the eye; treated by photocoagulation

PROTEINURIA protein in the urine, a sign of kidney damage; an earlier sign is microalbuminuria

RENAL THRESHOLD FOR GLUCOSE the kidney is more than a simple filter; it prevents glucose being lost in the urine until levels exceed a certain threshold, usually 8–10 mmol/l

SOLUBLE INSULIN unmodified insulin

SORBITOL a sugar formed from glucose by the enzyme aldose reductase; once formed it cannot get out of cells and causes them to swell; this is thought to be one mechanism underlying the formation of cataracts and neuropathy; sorbitol can be used as an artificial sweetener

STILBOESTROL a synthetic oestrogen or female hormone; it is still used in treating prostate cancer

SUBCUTANEOUS under the skin—the usual site for insulin injections

SULPHONYLUREAS a class of anti-diabetic tablets that work by increasing insulin release from the pancreas; examples include tolbutamide, chlorpropamide, glibenclamide, and glipizide

THIAZIDE DIURETICS a class of drugs that increase the production of urine; they also lower blood pressure

ULCER a long-standing breach in the skin

URAEMIA the illness resulting from retention of urea and other waste products in kidney failure

VASCULAR ENDOTHELIAL GROWTH FACTOR (VEGF) a family of proteins that are released by tissues in response to low oxygen levels; they increase the growth of small blood vessels (angiogenesis) and play a role in the development of diabetic retinopathy and spread of cancer

VASCULAR DISEASE disease affecting blood vessels

VITREOUS HUMOUR the jelly-like substance that fills the space between the lens of the eye and the retina

NOTES

Prologue

1. Simon Garfield, *Observer*, 29 July 2007, Comments and Features Section, p. 26.

2. United Nations General Assembly, *Resolution Adopted by the General Assembly – 61/225, World Diabetes Day*, New York: UN General Assembly, 2006.

3. Millimols per litre (mmol/l) is the Système Internationale (SI) unit of measurement used in Europe and most of the rest of the world. Americans express the concentration as milligrammes per decilitre (mg/dl). To convert mmol/l of glucose to mg/dl multiply by 18.

4. J. M. Malins, *Clinical Diabetes Mellitus* (London, 1968).

5. R. B. Tattersall, 'Mild familial diabetes with dominant inheritance', *Quarterly Journal of Medicine*, 43 (1974), 339–57.

6. R. Saundby, 'The modern treatment of diabetes mellitus', *Lancet*, 1 (1900), 1420–6.

Chapter 1

1. The papyrus was found in 1858 in Thebes by Georg Moritz Ebers. See R. H. Major, 'The Papyrus Ebers', *Annals of Medical History*, 2 (1930), 547–55.

2. C. L. Gemmill, 'The Greek concept of diabetes', *Bulletin of the New York Academy of Medicine*, 48 (1972), 1033–6.

3. E. J. Leopold, 'Aretaeus the Cappadocian', *Annals of Medical History*, 2 (1930), 424–35.

4. T. J. Hughes, *Thomas Willis 1621–1675: His Life and Work* (London, 1991).

5. Francis Home, *Clinical Experiments, Histories and Dissections* (Edinburgh, 1780).

6. John Rollo, *An Account of Two Cases of the Diabetes Mellitus: With Remarks, as They Arose during the Progress of the Cure to which Are Added, a General View of the Nature of the Disease and its Appropriate Treatment* (London, 1797).

7. John M. Camplin, *On Diabetes and its Successful Treatment* (London, 1858).

8. Quoted by Frederick Gowland Hopkins in 'Dr Pavy and diabetes', *Science Progess*, 7 (1912–13), 13–47. Hopkins, who later won a Nobel Prize for his discovery of vitamins, worked with Pavy as a medical student.

9. A. S. Donkin, 'Further observations on the skim-milk treatment of diabetes', *Lancet*, 1 (1873), 45–6.

10. W. Osler, *The Principles and Practice of Medicine* (New York, 1909), 421.

11. C. M. Durrant, 'Retrospective notes on outpatient practice', *BMJ*, 1 (1865), 245.

12. I have taken this translation from R. H. Major, *Classic Descriptions of Disease* (Springfield, Ill., 1978), 247–8.

13. F. W. Pavy, *Researches on the Nature and Treatment of Diabetes* (London, 1862), 220.

14. F. W. Pavy, 'Introductory address to the discussion on the clinical aspect of glycosuria', *Lancet*, 2 (1885), 1085–7.

15. F. W. Pavy, 'On diabetic neuritis', *Lancet*, 2 (1904), 71–3.

Chapter 2

1. C. H. Fagge and P. H. Pye-Smith, *A Textbook of Medicine* (London, 1901), 436.

2. W. Prout, *On the Nature and Treatment of Stomach and Renal Diseases* (5th edn, London, 1848), 23.

3. George Harley, *Diabetes: Its Various Forms and Different Treatments* (London, 1866).

4. Prout, *On the Nature and Treatment of Stomach and Renal Diseases*, 33.

5. R. Saundby, 'The modern treatment of diabetes mellitus', *Lancet*, 1 (1900), 1420–6, at p. 1421.

6. G. Laguesse, 'Sur la formation des îlots de Langerhans dans le pancréas', *C. R. Soc. Biol. Paris*, 46 (1894), 819–20.

7. C. E. Brown-Séquard, 'On a new therapeutic method consisting of the use of organic liquids extracted from glands and other organs', *BMJ*, 1 (1893), 1145–7, 1212–14, at p. 1213.

8. Editorial, 'Animal extracts as therapeutic agents', *BMJ*, 1 (1893), 1279.

9. E. A. Schäfer, 'On internal secretion', *BMJ*, 2 (1895), 342–8.

10. E. H. Starling, 'Croonian Lecture: on the chemical correlation of the functions of the body', *Lancet*, 2 (1905), 339–41, at p. 340.

11. Taken from an appreciation by Cornelia van Beek, 'Leonid. V. Sobolev, 1876–1919', *Diabetes*, 7 (1958), 245–8.

12. D. W. Richards, 'The effect of pancreas extract on depancreatised dogs: Ernest L. Scott's thesis of 1911', *Perspectives in Biology and Medicine*, 10 (1966), 84–95.

13. J. J. R. Macleod, *Physiology and Biochemistry in Modern Medicine* (3rd edn, London, 1921), 714.

14. A. E. Garrod, 'Lettsomian lectures on glycosuria', *Lancet*, 1 (1912), 483–8, at p. 485.

15. A. J. Hodgson, 'Diabetes mellitus', *Canadian Medical Association Journal*, 2 (1912), 874–91.

16. W. Osler, *The Principles and Practice of Medicine* (New York, 1909), 420.

17. Editorial '"Cures" for diabetes', *Lancet*, 2 (1915), 1207.

18. Alfred R. Henderson, 'Frederick M. Allen and the Physiatric [sic] Institute at Morristown, NJ', *Academy of Medicine of New Jersey Bulletin*, 16 (1970), 40–9.

19. G. Graham, 'The Goulstonian lectures on glycaemia and glycosuria', *Lancet*, 1 (1921), 1059–63.

20. E. P. Joslin, 'Present-day treatment and prognosis in diabetes', *American Journal of the Medical Sciences*, 150 (1915), 485–96.

21. O. Leyton, *Three Lectures on the Treatment of Diabetes Mellitus by Alimentary Rest (the 'Allen' Treatment)* (2nd edn, London, 1918).

22. J. R. Williams, 'An evaluation of the Allen method of treatment of diabetes mellitus', *American Journal of the Medical Sciences*, 162 (1921), 62–72.

23. F. J. Poynton, 'Five cases of diabetes mellitus in young children', *BMJ*, 1 (1923), 277–9.

Chapter 3

1. Quoted in M. Bliss, *The Discovery of Insulin* (Chicago, 1982), 50.

2. J. J. R. Macleod, 'History of the researches leading to the discovery of insulin [1922]', *Bulletin of the History of Medicine*, 52 (1978), 298–312.

3. F. G. Banting, C. H. Best, J. B. Collip, W. R. Campbell, and A. A. Fletcher, 'Pancreatic extracts in the treatment of diabetes mellitus: preliminary report', *Canadian Medical Association Journal*, 12 (1922), 141–6.

4. Quoted by M. Bliss, *Banting: A Biography* (Toronto, 1984).

5. M. Bliss, 'Rewriting medical history: Charles Best and the Banting and Best myth', *Journal of the History of Medicine*, 48 (1993), 253–74.

6. 'Canadian diabetes cure', *The Times*, 19 August 1922.

7. R. Carrasco-Formiguera, 'From the preinsulin age to the Banting and Best era: reminiscences of a witness and participant', *Israel Journal of Medical Sciences*, 8 (1972), 484–7.

8. 'Certain diabetes cure', *Nottingham Evening Post*, 20 April 1923.

9. 'A patient's point of view', *The Times*, 7 August 1923.

10. The part played by the MRC is described by Jonathan Liebenau, 'The MRC and the pharmaceutical industry: the model of insulin', in J. Austoker and L. Bryder (eds), *Historical Perspectives on the Role of the MRC: Essays in the History of the Medical Research Council of the United Kingdom and its Predecessor, the Medical Research Committee 1913–1953* (Oxford, 1989), 163–80.

11. Editorial, 'Reckless use of hypodermic injections', *Lancet*, 1 (1882), 358.

12. 'Report of meeting of Brighton and Sussex Medico-Chirugical Society', *BMJ*, 2 (1923), 765.

13. Quoted by F. I. R. Martin, *A History of Diabetes in Australia* (Victoria, 1998), 12.

14. E. P. Joslin, *The Treatment of Diabetes Mellitus* (4th edn, London, 1928), 81.

15. Carrasco-Formiguera, 'From the preinsulin age to the Banting and Best era'.

16. A. A. Fletcher and W. R. Campbell, 'The blood sugar following insulin administration and the symptom-complex hypoglycaemia', *Journal of Metabolic Research*, 2 (1922), 637–49.

17. E. P. Joslin, H. F. Root, and P. White, 'Diabetic coma and its treatment', *Medical Clinics of North America*, 8 (1925), 1873–1919.

18. J. K. Rennie, 'A year's experience of insulin', *Lancet*, 1 (1925), 811–15.

19. W. F. Talbert and J. Sharnick, *Playing for Life* (Boston and Toronto, 1958).

20. R. D. Lawrence and K. Madders, 'The employment of diabetics', *BMJ*, 2 (1938), 1076–7.

21. 'Diabetics at work or on holiday', repr. in *Diabetic Journal* (Dec. 1948), 301.

22. References for these obituaries can be found in R. B. Tattersall, 'A force of magical activity: the introduction of insulin treatment in Britain 1922–1926', *Diabetic Medicine*, 12 (1995), 739–55.

23. H. Droller, 'An outbreak of hepatitis in a diabetic clinic', *BMJ*, 1 (1945), 623–5.

24. E. A. M. Gale, 'Fifty years of type 1 diabetes', *British Journal of Diabetes and Vascular Disease*, 2 (2002), 441–5, at p. 443.

Chapter 4

1. All these quotations are taken from R. M. Wilder, 'Recollections and reflections on education, diabetes, other metabolic diseases, and nutrition in the Mayo clinic and associated hospitals, 1919–1950', *Perspectives in Biology and Medicine*, 1 (1958), 237–77.

2. C. M. Fletcher, 'One way of coping with diabetes', *BMJ*, 1 (1980), 1115–16.

3. L. Vargas, 'Subcutaneous implantation of insulin in diabetes mellitus', *Lancet*, 1 (1949), 598–601.

4. C. Feudtner, *Bittersweet: Diabetes, Insulin and the Transformation of Illness* (Chapel Hill, NC, 2003), 132–43.

5. E. Tolstoi, 'Newer concepts in the treatment of diabetes mellitus with protamine insulin', *American Journal of Digestive Diseases*, 10 (1943), 247–53.

6. F. M. Allen, 'Current judgments on metabolic control and complications in diabetes', *New England Journal of Medicine*, 248 (1953), 133–6.

7. R. T. Woodyatt, 'Psychic and emotional factors in general diagnosis and treatment', *Journal of the American Medical Association*, 89 (1927), 1013–14.

8. C. Feudtner and S. Gabbe, 'Diabetes and pregnancy: four motifs of modern medical history', *Clincal Obstetrics and Gynecology*, 43 (2000), 4–16.

9. J. W. Farquhar, 'The child of the diabetic woman', *Archives of Diseases of Childhood*, 34 (1959), 76–96.

Chapter 5

1. J. E. Poulsen, 'The Houssay phenomenon in man: recovery from retinopathy in a case of diabetes with Simmond's disease', *Diabetes*, 2 (1953), 7–12. The final course and post-mortem results are in *Diabetes*, 15 (1966), 73–7.

2. M. Ghavamian, C. Gutch, K. Kopp, and W. Kolff, 'The sad truth about haemodialysis in diabetic nephropathy', *Journal of the American Medical Association*, 222 (1971), 1386 9.

3. Anon., 'Any questions?', *BMJ*, 2 (1973), 167.

4. Quoted in D. E. R. Sutherland et al., 'Evolution of kidney, pancreas, and islet transplantation for patients with diabetes at the University of Minnesota', *American Journal of Surgery*, 166 (1993), 456–85.

5. J. M. Malins, *Clinical Diabetes Mellitus* (London, 1968), 171.

6. W. R. Jordan, 'Neuritic manifestations in diabetes mellitus', *Archives of Internal Medicine*, 57 (1936), 307–66.

7. R. W. Rundles, 'Diabetic neuropathy: general review with report of 125 cases', *Medicine (Baltimore)*, 24 (1945), 111–60.

8. M. Ellenberg, 'Diabetic neuropathic cachexia', *Diabetes*, 23 (1974), 418–23.

Chapter 6

1. S. Silbert, 'Mid-leg amputations for gangrene in the diabetic', *Annals of Surgery*, 127 (1948), 503–12.

2. E. P. Joslin, 'The menace of diabetic gangrene', *New England Journal of Medicine*, 211 (1934), 16–20.

3. W. W. Oakley, R. F. C. Caterall, and M. M. Martin, 'Aetiology and mangement of lesions of the feet in diabetes', *BMJ*, 2 (1956), 953–7.

4. P. Brand, *Insensitive Feet: A Practical Handbook on Foot Problems in Leprosy* (London, 1966).

5. P. Brand and P. Yancey, *Pain: The Gift Nobody Wants* (London, 1994), 182.

6. Joslin, 'The menace of diabetic gangrene'.

7. S. Strouse, 'Control methods in the treatment of diabetes mellitus', *Journal of the American Medical Association*, 75 (1920), 97–101.

8. E. Hinkle Lawrence Jr., 'Customs, emotions, and behavior in the dietary treatment of diabetes', *Journal of the American Dietetic Association*, 41 (1962), 341–4.

9. F. B. Peck Sen., 'Third Lilly Conference on Carbutamide', *Diabetes*, 6 (1957), 1.

10. Editorial statement, *Diabetes*, 19 (1970), supp., p. 747.

11. Editorial, 'Oral hypoglycaemics in diabetes mellitus', *Lancet*, 2 (1975), 489–91.

12. J. M. Moss, 'The UGDP scandal and cover-up', *Journal of the American Medical Association*, 232 (1975), 806–8.

Chapter 7

1. J. B. Walker, 'Field work of a diabetic clinic', *Lancet*, 2 (1953), 445–7.

2. W. Gepts, 'Pathologic anatomy of the pancreas in juvenile diabetes', *Diabetes*, 14 (1965), 619–33.

Chapter 8

1. G. F. Cahill, D. D. Etzwiler, and N. Freinkel, 'Control and diabetes', *New England Journal of Medicine*, 294 (1976), 1004–5.

2. R. B. Tattersall and E. A. M. Gale, 'Patient self-monitoring of blood glucose and refinements of conventional insulin treatment', *American Journal of Medicine*, 70 (1981), 177–82.

Chapter 9

1. R. Saundby, 'Diabetes mellitus', *Medical Annual* (Bristol, 1897), 675.

2. C. L. Bose, 'Discussion on diabetes in the tropics', *BMJ*, 2 (1907), 1051–64.

3. E. P. Joslin, L. I. Dublin, and H. H. Marks, 'Studies in diabetes mellitus: III. Interpretation of the variations in diabetes incidence', *American Journal of the Medical Sciences*, 189 (1935), 163–93.

4. E. Bulmer, 'The menace of obesity', *BMJ*, 1 (1932), 1024–6.

5. R. Tattersall, 'Diseases the doctor (or autoanalyser) says you have got', *Clinical Medicine*, 1 (2001), 230–3.

6. E. P. Joslin, 'Social and medical aspects of the problem of heredity', *Medical Clinics of North America*, 18 (1935), 1033–40, at pp. 1033–4, 1035.

7. J. V. Neel, S. S. Fajans, J. W. Conn, and R. T. Davidson, 'Diabetes mellitus', in J. V. Neel, M. W. Shaw, and W. J. Schull (eds), *The Genetics and Epidemiology of Chronic Diseases*, Public Health Service Publication No. 1163 (Washington, 1965).

8. G. M. Reaven, 'Role of insulin resistance in human disease– Banting lecture 1988', *Diabetes*, 37 (1988), 1595–1607.

Postscript

1. F. M. Allen, 'Personal view of therapy of diabetes mellitus', *Diabetes*, 11 (1962), 336–8.

2. C. M. Fletcher, 'Avoiding diabetic disabilities without loss of freedom', *Journal of the Royal College of Physicians*, 16 (1982), 78–9.

3. J. D. Eastwood, 'Insulin and Independence', *BMJ*, 293 (1986), 1659–61.

SUGGESTIONS FOR FURTHER READING

Prologue

To find out more about the medical aspects of diabetes, a good starting point would be one of the many patient handbooks. Ones that I think are particularly good are: Charles Fox and Anne Kilvert, *Type 2 Diabetes: Answers at your Fingertips* (London, 2007). A companion volume by the same authors deals with type 1. I would also recommend Rowan Hillson, *Diabetes Care, a Practical Manual* (Oxford, 2008), which is aimed at GPs, junior doctors, and specialist nurses.

As with any other subject, there is a plethora of information on the Internet. One site that I have found reliable is David Mendosa, www.mendosa.com.

Chapter 1

No general history of diabetes has been published since 1989. In fact, I know of only three before that; two short volumes, N. S. Papaspyros, *The History of Diabetes Mellitus* (London, 1952), Jacob E. Poulsen, *Features of the History of Diabetology* (Copenhagen, 1982), and a much more comprehensive one, Hans Schadewaldt, *Geschichte des Diabetes Mellitus* (Berlin, 1975), which is available only in German. Dietrich von Engelhardt,

Diabetes: Its Medical and Cultural History (Berlin, 1989), is a collection of reprinted essays and historical vignettes.

Chapter 2

Two biographies of Claude Bernard are J. M. D. Olmsted, *Claude Bernard: Physiologist* (London, 1939), F. L. Holmes, *Claude Bernard and Animal Chemistry* (Cambridge, Mass, 1974).

There is no full-length biography of Oskar Minkowski, although one is being written.

An authoritative account of the work of Brown-Séquard is Michael J. Aminoff, *Brown-Séquard: A Visionary of Science* (New York, 1993).

For more on the search for insulin, see R. B. Tattersall, 'Pancreatic organotherapy for diabetes 1889–1921' *Medical History*, 39 (1995), 288–316.

Chapter 3

The definitive account of how insulin was discovered is Michael Bliss, *The Discovery of Insulin* (Chicago, 1982). Bliss has also written the excellent *Banting: A Biography* (Toronto, 1984).

There is a website, www.discoveryofinsulin.com, which has photos of Banting and a copy of his Nobel lecture. A lot of original material can be accessed on line at the website of the Fisher Library of the University of Toronto, *http://digital.library.utoronto. ca/insulin*. It also includes recollections and pictures of some of Banting's original patients.

Good articles on insulin coma therapy are F. E. James, 'Insulin treatment in psychiatry', *History of Psychiatry*, 3 (1992), 221–35, and D. B. Doroshow, 'Performing a cure for schizophrenia: insulin coma therapy on the wards', *Journal of the Hisory of Medicine and Allied Sciences*, 62 (2007), 213–43.

Chapter 4

Torsten Deckert's *HC Hagedorn and Danish Insulin* (Copenhagen, 2000) is a very readable account of the invention of long-acting insulins and the rivalry between the two Danish insulin manufacturers.

Chris Feudtner, *Bittersweet: Diabetes, Insulin and the Transformation of Illness* (Chapel Hill, NC, 2003), explores the experience of complications in Joslin's patients through their correspondence with Joslin and his associates.

There is no easily accessible history of diabetic pregnancy, but the first four chapters in Moshe Hod et al. (eds), *Textbook of Diabetes and Pregnancy* (2nd edn, London, 2008), cover the history and the contributions of White and Pedersen.

Chapter 5

Andie Dominick, *Needles: A Memoir of Growing up with Diabetes.* (New York, 1998), is a poignant account of stuttering blindness from retinopathy.

Although not specifically about diabetes, a biography of Wilhelm Kolff by Jacob van Noordwijk, *Dialysing for Life* (Dordrecht, 2001), documents the development of the artificial kidney.

For further information about laser treatment, the NHS has produced a useful leaflet, 'Preparing for laser treatment for diabetic retinopathy and maculopathy'.

Chapter 6

The importance of pain sensation is explained in P. Brand and P. Yancey, *Pain: The Gift Nobody Wants* (London, 1994).

Chapter 7

There is no biography of Solomon Berson, but his work with Yalow is described in Eugene Straus, *Rosalyn Yalow: Her Life and Work in Medicine* (Cambridge, Mass., 1998). Georgina Ferry's *Dorothy Hodgkin: A Life* (Cambridge, 1998) is an engaging account of a remarkable woman. The Nobel Prize website, Nobelprize. org, has biographies of all Nobel prize winners, such as Fred Sanger, Dorothy Hodgkin, and Rosalyn Yalow. This website also has the prizewinners' speeches, in which they describe their work in detail. John Pickup and Harry Keen's 'Continuous subcutaneous insulin infusion at 25 years', *Diabetes Care*, 25 (2002), 593–8, can be accessed free on the Internet.

Chapter 8

As yet there is no history of either the DCCT or UKPDS. Further information about the UKPDS can be found on the website of the Diabetes Trials Unit of the University of Oxford, www.dtu. ox.ac.uk. Similar information for the DCCT is provided by the US National Diabetes Information Clearing House, www.diabetes.niddk.nih.gov/dm/pubs/control.

For an excellent account of the pros and cons of insulin analogues, see F. Holleman and E. A. M. Gale, 'Nice insulins, pity about the evidence', *Diabetologia*, 50 (2007), 1783–90.

Chapter 9

The International Diabetes Federation has produced a 'Diabetes Atlas', which reached its third edition in 2008 and is available free online at idf.org. It tells you everything you could wish to know about the epidemiology of diabetes in the twenty-first century.

Thomas Royle Dawber, *The Framingham Study* (Cambridge, Mass., 1980), is a description of the study by the main organizer.

For a sociological account of the Pimas, see Carolyn Smith-Morris, *Diabetes among the Pima: Stories of Survival* (Tuscon, 2006).

INDEX